QUICK GUIDE – COLOR CODED CHAPTERS

First Responder Press

Published by First Responder Press LLC
Bonsall, California

Copy Edited by Jacqueline Aussie

Available from Amazon.com and Other Retail Outlets

Available on Kindle and Other Devices

THE OFF-DUTY EMS MANUAL FOR IN-FLIGHT MEDICAL EMERGENCIES

ISBN-10: 0-9988016-0-7 ISBN-13: 978-0-9988016-0-5

THE OFF-DUTY EMS MANUAL FOR IN-FLIGHT MEDICAL EMERGENCIES

First Responder Press

www.FirstResponderPress.com

Adam Daniel Chase, EMT, MPS

This Manual Belongs to:	
Name:	
Badge/I.D.:	Phone:
Department Name:	
If found, please return to the address listed below:	
Address:	
E-Mail:	

PREFACE

As an Emergency Medical Services (EMS) professional for over two decades, I recognize *The Off-Duty EMS Manual for In-Flight Medical Emergencies* satisfies a real need in modern airline safety. The majority of airlines focus on "doctors" or "physicians" when planning for the next in-flight medical emergency (IFME), but there is another class of medical professional that can attend to patients in-flight, they are off-duty EMS professionals. These off-duty EMS professionals consist of paramedics, firefighters, and emergency medical technicians (EMTs). These professionals are 911 first responders who already answer the call for help, anywhere and at any time, making them ideal for IFMEs.

The purpose of this manual is to provide these off-duty EMS professionals with a guideline of best practices for the most common IFMEs. In addition, this manual also provides specific answers to common questions and concerns that may be asked before, during, and after an IFME. Important procedures such as contacting ground-based physicians through a company called "MedAire" will be highlighted for easy instruction during an emergency. This manual is designed to be thorough and easy to navigate during an IFME.

This manual is intended to be used by off-duty EMS professionals who would be covered under the Aviation Medical Assistance Act's Good Samaritan Provision and/or similar international laws. Although any person may attend to and/or help care for a passenger during an IFME, the Good Samaritan law only covers those individuals trained and certified to administer medical treatment (House of Representatives, 1998).

This manual lists the required medical equipment airlines are mandated to carry aboard all domestic and international flights. The off-duty EMS professionals using this manual will find itemized lists for all the required medical equipment stowed for flight. As per international and domestic law, all airlines are responsible for providing and maintaining their specific emergency medical equipment. This manual is a supplement to the mandated emergency medical kit (EMK). It is recommended that off-duty EMS professionals review this manual prior to traveling. The medical training provided in this manual may serve as continuing education credits if approved by the user's respective agency. Agencies that send their employees for training by commercial airlines outside their local jurisdiction should provide a copy of this manual and recommend the reviewing of this manual prior to travel.

The leaders in airline safety are the men, women, and companies that take pride in improving aircraft safety, emergency equipment, and procedures prior to FAA mandates. We congratulate the Lufthansa Group, Turkish Airlines, and the ANA Group who have all recently implemented a volunteer "Doctors on Board" service within their fly mile programs. After reviewing this manual, readers should agree that all airlines shall implement similar services and not just for doctors, but for the EMS community as well. Doctors are not always around at 30,000 feet, airlines should implement an "EMS & Doctors on Board" program to successfully reach more medical professionals during the next IFME!

SPECIAL THANKS AND DEDICATIONS

Adam D. Chase would like to thank those individuals that helped make this manual possible. Hundreds of hours of research and analysis went into this manual. Penn State professor James F. McKenzie, PhD, MPH empowered Chase through scholarly research to create the *Off-Duty EMS Manual for In-Flight Medical Emergencies*. The wonderful staff at the Penn State Graduate Writing Center spent hours with Chase on one-on-one writing consultations related to this manual. Chase would like to thank Attorney Brandy Karl, the Penn State Copyright Officer for reviewing this manual and answering questions related to copyright and fair use. Chase would like to thank his wife Millie Chase, his family, and friends for reviewing and commenting on the multiple drafts of this manual. Chase is very grateful for Jacqueline Aussie and her professional editing experience related to the medical industry, she copy-edited this manual.

This manual is dedicated to the off-duty EMS professionals (paramedics, EMTs, firefighters), lifeguards, park rangers, medically trained law enforcement, and related medical professionals who without hesitation, will be rendering medical assistance during the next IFME.

Adam Daniel Chase, EMT, MPS, has worked as a first responder in Southern California for over twenty-five years. He is a certified emergency medical technician and serves in middle management as a municipal park police officer.

Chase recently graduated from the Penn State College of Medicine, where he earned his master of professional studies degree in homeland security and public health preparedness. Chase also completed a graduate certificate in public health with an emphasis on bioterrorism and disaster preparedness. He received his bachelor's degree in public administration with an emphasis on law enforcement from Upper Iowa University.

Chase has always been interested in airline safety. Now he has combined his education and experience to provide the first manual specifically designed for off-duty medical personnel facing an in-flight medical emergency.

TABLE OF CONTENTS

LIST OF TABLES & FIGURES

ACRONYMS & ABBREVIATIONS USED IN THIS MANUAL

24/7, 24 Hours per Day, Seven Days a Week

AED, Automated External Defibrillator

AFAK, Aircraft First Aid Kit

ALS, Advanced Life Support

AMA, Against Medical Advice

AMAA, Aviation Medical Assistance Act of 1998

BLS, Basic Life Support

BP, Blood Pressure

BVM, Bag Valve Mask

C, Centigrade or Celsius

CC, Cubic Centimeter

CFR, Code of Federal Regulations

CPR, Cardiopulmonary Resuscitation

CO2, Carbon Dioxide

Combitube, Tracheal-Esophageal Combitube Airway

CVA, Cerebral Vascular Accident

DEA, Drug Enforcement Administration

DNR, Do Not Resuscitate

Dx, Diagnosis

EASA, European Aviation Safety Agency

ECC, Emergency Cardiac Care

ECG or **EKG**, Electrocardiogram

ED, Emergency Department

EMK, Emergency Medical Kit

EMS, Emergency Medical Services

EMT, Emergency Medical Technician

EMT-P, Emergency Medical Technician - Paramedic

EEMK, Enhanced Emergency Medical Kit – same as **XMK**, Expanded Medical Kit

ER, Emergency Room

ETT, Endotracheal Tube

ExDS, Excited Delirium

F, Fahrenheit

FAA, Federal Aviation Administration

FAK, First Aid Kit (Aviation)

First Call (The), Ground-Based Airline Physicians & an International SOS Company Based in Scotland

GI, Gastrointestinal

HR, Heart Rate

IATA, International Air Transport Association

ICAO, International Civil Aviation Organization

IFME, In-Flight Medical Emergency

IV, Intravenous

IFME, In-Flight Medical Emergency

JAA, Joint Aviation Authorities

JAA-TO, Joint Aviation Authorities Training Organization

King Tube, King Tube LTS Single Use Supraglottic Airway

LPM, Liters per Minute

Luftsicherheitsgesetz, Airline Captain - Equivalent Enforcement Powers of Policeman

MedAire, Ground-Based Airline Physicians & an International SOS Company

MedLink, 24-hr Telemedicine Center Provided by MedAire

MG, Milligram

ML, Milliliter

NTSB, National Transportation Safety Board

O_2, Medical Oxygen

PT, Patient

PTC, Patient Transport Compartment

PTU NG, Patient Transport Unit Next Generation

RN, Registered Nurse

Rx, Prescription, Treatment

S/S, Signs and Symptoms

STAT-MD, 24-hr Telemedicine Center Provided by the University of Pittsburgh Medical Center

Syncope, Fainting

UPK, Universal Precaution Kit

XMK, Expanded Medical Kit – same as EEMK

AN INTRODUCTION TO IN-FLIGHT MEDICAL EMERGENCIES

Are you prepared for this announcement: "This is your Captain speaking, is there a medical professional on-board? If so, please notify a flight attendant." In the event, there were off-duty Emergency Medical Service (EMS) professionals on-board the flight, the chances are they would not be prepared to handle a medical emergency, especially if they have not read this manual. In many cases, the off-duty EMS professionals aboard commercial flights are passengers (on vacation or professional travel) and would most likely have the mindset: "there must be another Emergency Medical Technician (EMT) or physician onboard to handle the call for help." Unfortunately, this is not always the case and it is important to remember that one medically trained individual is always better than none. Research suggests that there are many occasions when there are no medically trained professionals on board during any given flight; the chance of having a physician among the passengers has been reported to be as low as 40% (Brennan, 2013; Buchanan, Duong, Katzer, Memmer, & Weber, 2014). When adding off-duty EMS professionals to the above equation, research suggests the percentage doubles to nearly 80% (Peterson et al., 2013). This manual will introduce readers/users to the knowledge needed for an off-duty EMS professional to feel comfortable responding to medical emergencies aboard any commercial flight. This manual shall also highlight the fact that off-duty EMS professionals are more involved with airline related medical emergencies than data indicates.

With nearly 2.75 billion commercial airline passengers annually, the number of in-flight medical emergencies (IFMEs) continues to rise, yet the medical response to these IFMEs is dependent upon volunteers (Peterson et al., 2013). All U.S. and international commercial airlines primarily rely upon their passengers to provide basic-to-advanced medical care during IFMEs. These medically trained passengers are generally off-duty EMS professionals such as paramedics, firefighters, and EMTs. In the United States alone, requests from commercial airline flight crews for IFMEs are made approximately 50 times per day (Bashir, 2014). Although 50 domestic IFMEs per day may seem like a large number, it is not. On average, there are 28,537 daily U.S. commercial flights which equates to medical emergencies occurring for 1 out of nearly 600 flights (National Oceanic and Atmosphere Administration [NOAA], 2015; Peterson et al.). When factoring in intercontinental flights, the number of IFME increases to 1 in every 10,000 to 40,000 passengers resulting in a 98% probability that an IFME will occur in 1 of every 26 intercontinental flights; if each of these flights contain 400 or more passengers (Graf, Stuben, & Pump, 2012). The IFME odds go up dramatically when factoring in new generation mega-aircraft such as the Airbus A380-900 which has a maximum passenger capacity of 853 (Airbus, 2015). The Lufthansa registry further supports this claim, indicating that 70% of its airlines IFMEs occurred on long-haul intercontinental flights (Graf, Stuben, & Pump, 2012). When comparing commuter flights to intercontinental flights, there are fewer reported incidents of IFMEs primarily due to passenger capacity and flight durations. During a recent interview with a U.S. airline pilot, Captain Ian Stocke, his recall of IFMEs was rare, stating that IFMEs occurred approximately two times over a period of approximately 2,500 piloted flights. Overall, Peterson et al. revealed that approximately 44,000 IFMEs occur around the world annually.

PURPOSE OF THIS MANUAL

The primary purpose of this manual is to prepare the off-duty EMS professional for the most common IFMEs they may encounter while in-flight. The secondary purpose of this manual is to better prepare physicians and nurses who may be working alongside off-duty EMS professionals during the next IFME incident. Because off-duty EMS professionals handle more types of emergency calls on a regular basis when compared to general physicians, it is important that physicians realize that they may not be able to offer the best IFME care when compared to off-duty EMS professionals. A responding physician "should be willing to cede care of the patient to someone who has more experience" (Stewart, Agin, & Douglas, 2013, p. 1775) even if this means allowing an EMT to handle the IFME.

Previously, it has been believed that physicians have responded to the majority of IFMEs, but data now suggests this claim may not entirely be true (Sand, Bechara, Sand, & Mann, 2009). It is believed that off-duty EMS professionals play a bigger role today on IFMEs than previously believed, as much as 10 times what current data suggests. The goal of this manual is to bring attention to the medical community that off-duty EMS professionals are ideal first responders for IFMEs. Peterson et al. (2013) concluded "we believe that airline passengers who are health care professionals should be aware of their potential role as volunteer responders to in-flight medical emergencies" (p. 2079). This manual builds upon this recommendation to address the most common questions, concerns, and legal requirements an off-duty EMS professional may have before, during, and after an IFME.

WHY IS THERE A NEED FOR THIS MANUAL?

During the early days of commercial airlines travel, transportation by air was reserved for very special occasions with every seat being a first-class seat. Flight attendants during this era were highly qualified to respond to medical emergencies in-flight, as they were all trained nurses (Graf et al., 2012). As technology, has changed over the last several decades, there has been less of an emphasis on medical training and more on lifesaving equipment. Currently, there is very little emergency medical training given to commercial airline crew members which is why there is such a need for off-duty EMS professionals on-board these flights. The flight crew's lack of training can be attributed to the lack of aviation legal requirements. According to a Federal Aviation Administration (FAA) (2006) document regarding the medical training of airline crews, only the following categories of medical training are required:

- Emergency Medical Equipment Location, Function, and Intended Operation
- Emergency Medical Event Coordination Among Aircraft Crew
- Emergency Medical Kit (EMK) Contents and "No Go" Items in the Kit
- Initial Instruction and Recurrent Instruction (Every 24 Months) on CPR and Automated External Defibrillator (AED) Use

Other countries may have different standards in terms of crewmember IFME training. Lufthansa, for example, requires a first aid course of 16 hours to be taken by their flight attendants (Graf et al., 2012). Still, 16 hours of first aid training is no comparison to the training of an off-duty EMS professional.

Due to the limited first-aid training of modern flight crews, commercial airline companies have relied heavily on the good-will of off-duty EMS professionals when medical emergencies occur in-flight. The FAA agrees and has required EMKs on most commercial aircraft since 1986 (Thompson, 2015).

The current required EMK is well-equipped with many tools and medications that an off-duty EMS professional may use in the field. In addition to the EMK, most commercial aircraft carry AEDs and portable oxygen tanks. This manual covers topics that would normally present themselves to the responding off-duty EMS professional during an IFME.

THE FIRST IN-FLIGHT MANUAL FOR OFF-DUTY EMS PROFESSIONALS

A thorough search of MEDLINE revealed that there was a gap in training between the commercial airline companies and the off-duty EMS professionals aboard their flights. The search resulted in no published documents related to manuals designed for off-duty EMS professionals and IFMEs. This manual will be the first manual designed specifically for off-duty EMS professional involved in IFMEs.

OFF-DUTY EMS PROFESSIONALS BEST SUITED FOR AN IN-FLIGHT MEDICAL EMERGENCY

When a call to 911 is made, EMS professionals responded to the call for help, anywhere, anytime, and all while risking their lives to save others. Although EMS professionals do not have the same medical training and knowledge as physicians, these medical professionals do have the expertise and training in dealing with medical emergencies outside the emergency department (ED), making these EMS professional ideal for IFMEs. Data from a University of Pittsburgh study, presented in Table 1 shows that off-duty EMS professionals involved in IFMEs had the highest percentage of patients admitted to local hospitals which highlights their importance in-flight, especially when treating life-threatening illnesses. This study shows that off-duty EMS professionals are more involved with critically ill patients when compared to physicians, nurses, and flight crews.

Table 1: IFME Hospitalization Rates of Passengers Per Type of Medical Volunteer (Highest to Lowest)		
1)	**Off-Duty EMS Professionals**	**10.2%**
2)	Physicians	9.3%
3)	Nurses	8.7%
4)	Flight Crew Only – No Passenger Volunteers	4.7%

Table 1, IFME Hospitalization Rates of Passengers, Source: Peterson et al., 2013

However, when comparing the number and type of medical professionals who respond to these IFMEs, the data appears to be overwhelmingly biased towards physicians (Table 2). Although the medical care provided by off-duty EMS professionals accounted for the highest number of hospital admitted IFME patients, Peterson et al. (2013) indicated that physicians provided the majority of IFME assistance at 48.1% when compared to off-duty EMS professionals at 4.4% (Table 2). This IFME data appears to be inaccurate.

Table 2: IFME On-Board Assistance Provided by Medical Professional Type (Highest to Lowest)		
1)	Physicians	48.1%
2)	Missing Data or No Medical Help Available	23.7%
3)	Nurses	20.1%
4)	**Off-Duty EMS Professionals**	**4.4%**
5)	Other Health Care Professionals	3.7%

Table 2, IFME On-Board Assistance, Source: Peterson et al., 2013

The fact that the Peterson et al. (2013) study showed such a variation between these two categories of medical professionals pertaining to: 1) their rate of hospital admitted IFME patients, and 2) their participation in IFMEs, suggested that the data collected by the airlines which was relayed to the ground-based physician service was either incomplete or biased towards the number of physicians involved in IFMEs. Interesting, it is well documented by Sand et al. (2009) that airlines do not routinely record IFME incidents. Additionally, the Peterson et al. study indicated that the number of non-physician's responding to IFMEs included other health care professionals as displayed in Table 2, making that total number of non-physicians (EMS, Nurses, Other) closer to 28%. This study still does not explain why off-duty EMS professionals accounted for only 4.4% of IFME responses but had the greatest number of admitted hospital patients when compared to physicians and nurses. For this reason, it is highly probable that there was a significant percentage of off-duty EMS professionals that were mistakenly categorized as physicians within the available IFME data. Currently, there is no uniform method for airlines to collect IFME data.

AIRLINE RECORDS INACCURATELY REPORT PERCENTAGE OF PHYSICIAN ASSISTANCE IN-FLIGHT

"Worldwide, it has been reported that only 17% of all IFMEs are documented, most inconsistently" (Sand et al., 2009, p. 3) and when researchers attempt to obtain data from the airline companies, the airlines are reluctant to share (Sand et al.).

The lack of consistent and accurate record keeping by the airlines shows there is a high likelihood airlines might be improperly classifying many off-duty EMS professionals as physicians. This is a likely scenario because an EMT-P (Paramedic) can start intravenous (IVs) treatment and administer drugs much like a physician, possibly giving an inaccurate impression to the flight crew that the EMT-P is a medical doctor. If airlines are not accurately tracking IFMEs, how are they tracking who worked on the patients?

Additionally, when inspecting what appears to be accurate airline records for IFMEs, data is often left out regarding the level of volunteer medical experience on-board. According to the Lufthansa registry, approximately 80% of IFMEs were treated by a physician or another medical professional such as a nurse or emergency medical technician (Graf et al., 2012). Based on the interpreted data, physicians are not separated from other medical professionals bolstering the point that off-duty EMS professionals are probably more involved with IFMEs than currently believed. It was also reported in the Lufthansa registry that only 50% of the physicians who were involved with an IFME filled out medical emergency cards to report the incident, further showing evidence of missing data (Graf et al.).

Since airlines are not required to record data on IFMEs and hospitals are required to document admitted patients (for care and insurance purposes), more weight in this study should be focused on the numbers attained from hospital records, indicating 10.2% of admitted patients (the largest group) were assisted in-flight by off-duty EMS professionals. It is believed that off-duty EMS professionals participate in far more IFMEs than currently believed, as much as 10 times the current recorded numbers of 4.4%. It shall also be noted that of the various studies conducted on IFMEs, none of the studies investigated the possibilities that more than one rescuer was involved with each IFME (e.g. firefighter, EMT, physician, all on-scene). During most medical aid calls within United States, a fire engine and an ambulance are dispatched, resulting in a minimum of at least three firefighters and one EMT-P on-scene. It is highly unlikely that for the majority of IFMEs, there is only one off-duty EMS professional or physician present. A global IFME database is needed to correct this problem, specifically with reporting the number of IFME volunteers and their certifications/qualifications per incident.

GOALS OF THIS MANUAL

- To explain regulations pertaining to off-duty EMS care and the Good Samaritan Law.
- List the contents of the EMK and the mandated medical equipment required by airlines.
- List the medications within the various medical kits.
- To provide off-duty medical professionals with the in-flight knowledge to care for patients safely and effectively during medical emergencies on commercial aircraft.
- To explain the authority of the captain and crew in-flight.
- To explain the process used to contact airline physicians in-flight through MedAire.
- To introduce the off-duty EMS professional to cabin air quality and pressure.
- To list the potential medical problems and dangers that are most likely to occur during a commercial flight that will require in-flight patient care.
- To list the top 10 IFMEs.
- Explain the process to divert an aircraft.
- Handling the death of a passenger in-flight.

INTENDED AUDIENCE

This manual was created primarily for use by off-duty EMS professionals (paramedics, EMTs, firefighters), lifeguards, park rangers, medically trained law enforcement, and related medical professionals who are qualified and willing to volunteer and help during an in-flight medical emergency. In addition to those mentioned, the secondary audience would be educational institutions, medical schools, physicians, FAA medical advisors, airline administrators, flight attendants, commercial pilots, airport fire/rescue personnel, and manufactures of in-flight medical products including the EMK/EEMK and AEDs.

HOW TO USE THIS MANUAL

The manual is intended to serve both as a quick reference guide during an actual IFME and provide thorough information for the off-duty EMS professional who may be traveling by commercial aircraft in the near future. The format of this manual will follow a color-coded chapter system. For real-time updates to this manual, please check www.firstresponderpress.com and click on the manual updates link.

Notes

Notes

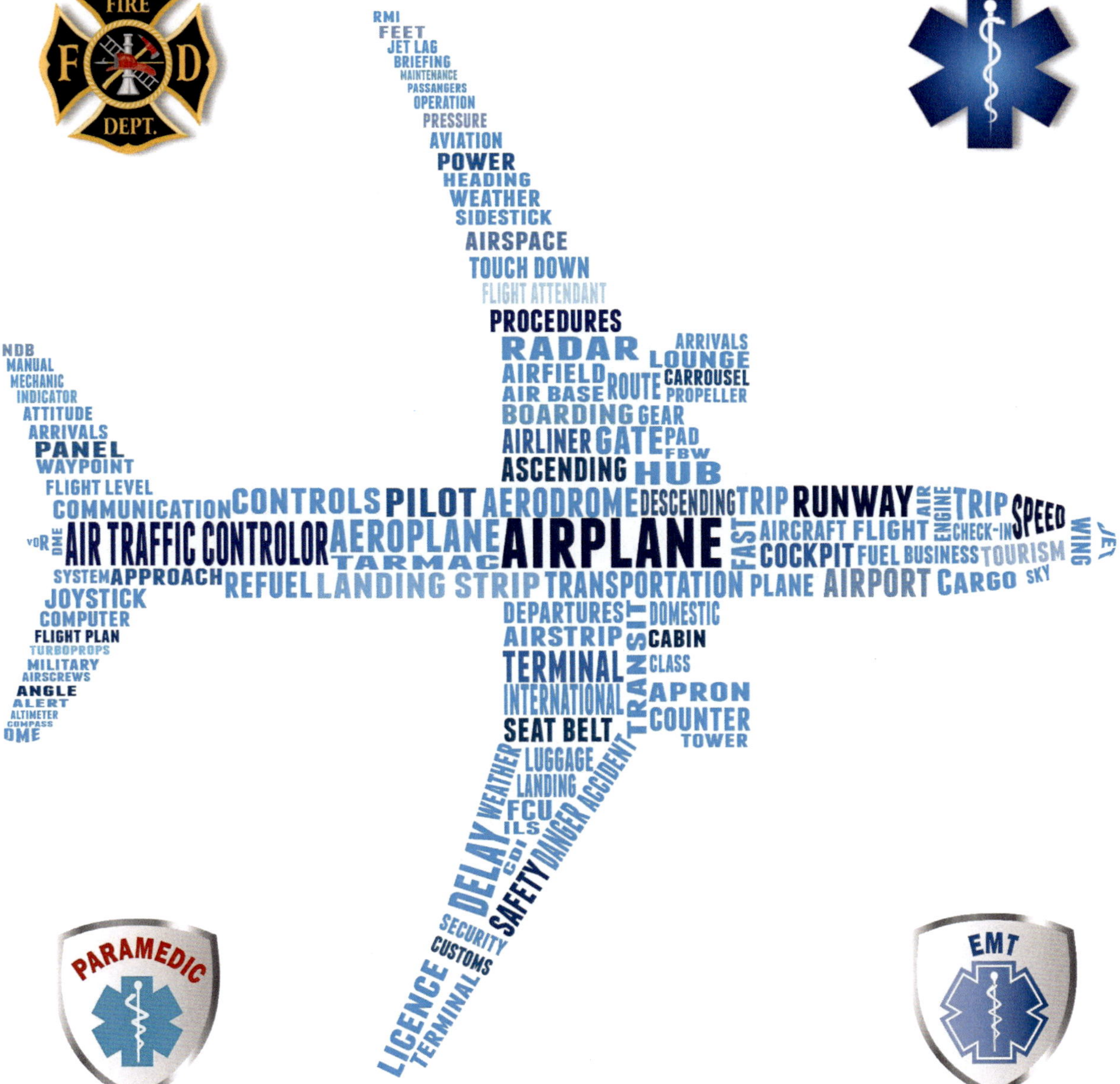

CHAPTER 1

Aviation Laws for Off-Duty EMS Professionals

CHAPTER 1: HIGHLIGHTS – AVIATION LAWS FOR OFF-DUTY EMS PROFESSIONALS

- **The Aviation Medical Assistance Act of 1998**
  - **U.S. Certified and Trained Medical Professionals According to Regulation**
    - ☑ Includes Physicians, Nurses, Paramedics, and Emergency Medical Technicians
    - ☑ Persons Who Are Licensed, Certified, or Qualified to Perform Medical Care
    - ☑ Good Samaritans when Requested by Crew
- **Off-Duty EMS Professional May Render Medical Treatment During an IFME**
  - ☑ No Oversight by Physicians Required
  - ☑ May Coordinate with Ground-Based Physicians and/or the Captain of the Aircraft
  - ☑ The Good Samaritan Provision
  - ☑ Off-Duty EMS Professionals are Under No Obligation to Respond to an IFME
- **International Laws are Similar to the U.S. FAA Laws**
  - ☑ Persons from Another Country That Hold a Valid Medical License or Certification
  - ☑ Airspace Above Territory Equals Country's Territory
  - ☑ Law of the Flag
  - ☑ Countries Requiring IFME Medical Intervention
  - ☑ Uniqueness of the Aviation Medical Assistance Act

1-1. THE AVIATION MEDICAL ASSISTANCE ACT OF 1998

- **The Aviation Medical Assistance Act of 1998** – Any State-qualified off-duty EMS professional is protected by the "Good Samaritan" provision against liability when involved with an IFME.
- **Good Samaritan Provision** - Off-duty EMS professionals can render same care that their training allows anywhere in the nation / world while in-flight on a U.S. registered airline.
- **No Physician Oversight Required** – Physician oversight is not practical in all circumstances and treatment may be provided regardless of the presence of a ground-based physician.
- **There is No U.S. Law Requiring Care** – From off-duty EMS professionals in-flight.

Aware of the limited medical resources available to passengers on commercial aircraft, in 1998 the U.S. Congress, in cooperation with the Federal Aviation Administration (FAA), passed the Aviation Medical Assistance Act to ensure medically trained volunteers including off-duty EMS professionals would have protections from legal liability if they rendered medical care in-flight (Peterson et al., 2013). Prior to 1998, there were no FAA regulations that offered liability protection to off-duty EMS or medical professionals. With the implementation of the Aviation Medical Assistance Act of 1998 (AMAA) came the "Good Samaritan" provision which protects an individual to include the passenger, pilot, and flight attendant from state and federal legal liability when helping during an IFME (House of Representatives, 1998). Under the Aviation Medical Assistance Act, "there is no obligation under Federal law to provide medical assistance to passengers" (Federal Aviation Administration, 2006, p. 4).

Outside the United States, laws are similar and most airlines are not required to provide medical care to their passengers, they are only required to provide certain medical kits and equipment (Peterson et al., 2013). The AMAA shall not be confused with the laws of other nations which may require off-duty EMS professionals or physicians to administer care.

1-1-1. THE GOOD SAMARITAN PROVISION OF THE AVIATION MEDICAL ASSISTANCE ACT OF 1998

The AMAA Good Samaritan Provision states:

> "An individual shall not be liable for damages in any action brought in a Federal or State court arising out of the acts or omissions of the individual in providing or attempting to provide assistance in the case of an in-flight medical emergency unless the individual, while rendering such assistance, is guilty of gross negligence or willful misconduct" (House of Representatives, 1998, p. 4).

This provision also states that the airline will have immunity from liability if: 1) the passenger was not an airline employee and 2) the airline crew believed in good faith that the passenger rendering aid was a medically qualified individual (House of Representatives, 1998).

1-1-2. DEFINED – MEDICALLY TRAINED INDIVIDUAL

The term "**medically trained individual**" pertaining to off-duty EMS professionals is defined as:

> "Any persons who is licensed, certified, or otherwise qualified to provide medical care in a State, including a physician, nurse, physician assistant, paramedic, and emergency medical technician" (House of Representatives, 1998, p. 3).

1-1-3. ABANDONMENT OF CARE LIABILITY

Unlike state observed laws which prohibit the off-duty EMS professional's abandonment of care during emergency medical incidents, there is no such regulation for IFMEs when aboard U.S. operated aircraft. There may be situations in-flight when off-duty EMS professionals are not mentally prepared or otherwise unable to continue care after initially responding to the call for help. When an off-duty EMS professional decides to help during an IFME, there is no obligation to continue care and there is no abandonment liability if the off-duty EMS professional ceases treatment (House of Representatives, 1998).

1-1-4. REQUIREMENT TO SHOW FLIGHT CREW IDENTIFICATION / CREDENTIALS

Each airline is responsible for providing their flight crews with policy on requesting the identification/medical credentials of medically trained passengers prior to their involvement with an IFME (Liao, 2010). The airlines requirement may include:

- The employer issued EMS professional identification card
- The State issued medical credential certificate or card
- County/City issued medical credentials
- Employer business card indicating medical certification

Note: EMS National Registry – "National Certification is NOT a license to practice. For specific licensing information contact the state in which you wish to practice" (State EMS agency information, 2015, para. 1).

Flight attendants may prefer to keep a business card with the off-duty EMS professional's medical classification indicated on the card, this will help the flight crew properly document the IFME incident indicating the level of care provided. In some cases, flight crews cannot confirm an off-duty EMS professional's qualifications due to their lack of credentials. During these situations where no credentials are presented, an off-duty EMS professional's qualifications may be taken on trust (Cocks & Liew, 2007). If there is a conflict between the flight crew's approval of an off-duty EMS professional's qualifications, the captain of the plane makes the final decision.

1-1-5. CANNOT RECEIVE PAYMENT FOR SERVICES

To be protected under the laws within the United States and internationally, an off-duty EMS professional cannot receive or expect to receive a payment for their services (Cocks & Liew, 2007). After an IFME incident, an airline may offer the affected off-duty EMS professional award points to a frequent flyer program, offer complimentary beverages and meals in-flight, or offer a seat upgrade to first class.

1-2. INTERNATIONAL LAWS PERTAINING TO IN-FLIGHT MEDICAL EMERGENCIES

Like U.S. FAA regulations, international airlines are not required to provide medical assistance or provide medically-trained personnel to handle IFMEs. The only exception to this rule is that airlines must attempt to locate a medically-trained professional on-board the flight to assist with an emergency (Peterson et al., 2013). All commercial airlines rely on off-duty EMS professionals because it would be extremely costly to outfit regular flights with on-board medical staff. Interestingly, some airlines choose to offer flight attendants more first aid training than others. Lufthansa currently requires a 16 hour first aid course for its flight attendants (Gabel et al., 2011).

Unlike the United States, some countries require physicians and off-duty EMS professionals to assist with IFMEs occurring over their specific territory; medically trained passengers who fail to assist can be held criminally liable if the aircraft lands within one of these defined territories, such as Germany or Australia (Gabel et al., 2011). To ensure uniformity within the European airspace, the Joint Aviation Authorities (JAA) was formed much like the U.S. based FAA for dealing with regulations pertaining to air travel. In fact, "much emphasis was placed on harmonizing the JAA regulations with those of the USA" (Joint Aviation Authorities, 2009, para. 1). Many emergency related equipment on-board U.S. and European flights are certified as both FAA and JAA compliant. In 2002, however, the European Aviation Safety Agency (EASA) was created to better control the EU regulatory and executive duties of the civilian aviation industry, taking over many of the tasks for which the JAA was previously responsible for (European Aviation Safety Industry, 2015).

1-2-1. EUROPEAN JOINT AVIATION AUTHORITY & EUROPEAN AVIATION SAFETY AGENCY

The JAA had 34 European members and was established to harmonize the legal policies and procedures for the European airline industry including the operation and maintenance of the passenger aircraft (Gabel et al., 2011). Recently, before its disbandment in 2009, the JAA served several functions under EASA, there was a Liaison and Training Office that was known as JAA-T for "transition" (Joint Aviation Authorities,

2009). Today, the JAA-T exists with 43 members under EASA as a co-operation, primarily for training. EASA is now the primary aviation authority for Europe to ensure the safety of all air travel.

1-2-1-1. International Laws for In-Flight Medical Emergencies

When an aircraft is in-flight, "flag right" or "law of the flag" are in effect. "Flag right" or "law of the flag" pertaining to in-flight aircraft, carries the international understanding that "the applicable laws are those of the country under whose jurisdiction the aircraft or airline operates" (Graf et al., 2012, p. 595). Flag rights usually pertain to the country or aviation authority where the aircraft is registered with one exception, when the plane is on the ground (Cocks & Liew, 2007). For example, a flight from Germany to the United States on a United Airlines aircraft, would have flag rights in the United States and would therefore be subject to FAA regulations and U.S. laws. On the other hand, a Lufthansa flight from Germany to the United States would have flag rights under the Federal Republic of Germany and therefore be subject to EASA regulations and German laws. The complicated part of this equation is when one of these flights diverts for a medical emergency to a foreign country, the laws of that territory can be applied when the plane is on the ground.

1-2-1-2. International Law - Physician Requirements

Several countries such as Germany, France, Australia, and the Middle East have laws that explicitly require physicians at the scene of a medical emergency to render aid or be subject to arrest and financial penalties (Graf et al., 2012). These laws are not specific to air travel, but do apply to IFMEs when the aircraft's or airlines flag right is from one of these countries. If an aircraft flies over a territory that has specific laws related to the requirement of rendering medical aid, generally the law pertains to the aircrafts flag rights and not the country that the plane flew over. Additionally, these laws primarily focus on physicians but may affect all medical professionals including off-duty EMS professionals.

Note: When in doubt, contact MedLink or ground-based service for advice from a physician.

1-2-1-3. International Good Samaritan Laws

Many countries have Good Samaritan laws on the ground but the United States is the only country that specifically offers volunteer medical professionals immunity from legal action from state and federal courts. "Many airlines indemnify doctors who volunteer, and will offer written confirmation from the aircraft captain of this, if the doctor requests it" (Cocks & Liew, 2007, p. 5). The same should apply for off-duty EMS professionals, but always ask the flight crew for clarification.

1-2-1-4. When International In-Flight Medical Treatment Goes Wrong

At times, mentally unstable passengers may become unruly and need to be restrained. Some of these passengers may be suffering from unknown medical conditions or be under the influence of alcohol and/or drugs. Care must be taken in situations where medical intervention may make a situation worse, especially when the aircraft's flag rights are unknown to the off-duty EMS professional. In 1999, an unruly airline passenger was given an IV sedation by a physician in-flight and as a result, died. When the plane landed, Turkish authorities arrested the flight crew and the physician (Cocks & Liew, 2007). Lord Justice Stuart-Smith said this well when describing the duty of a volunteer doctor, "his only duty as a matter of law is to not make the victim's condition worse" (Cocks & Liew, 2007). The best treatments are sometimes the least invasive and in the above example, restraining the passenger with handcuffs or other restraints would have been sufficient to control the unruly passenger.

1-3. DOCTORS ON BOARD PROGRAM

Physicians and off-duty EMS professionals all over the world may be reluctant to volunteer during an IFME for several reasons. To help encourage doctors (specifically physicians) to participate during IFMEs, several airlines including Lufthansa, Turkish, and ANA have begun implementing programs. Unfortunately, as airlines roll out these new IFME programs, they forget about the EMS community. IFME data indicates that doctors are only available 40% of the time, the airlines need to address this issue and add EMS professionals to their programs!

1-3-1. LUFTHANSA DOCTORS ON BOARD PROGRAM

In 2006, Lufthansa Airlines developed a "Doctor on Board" program for both Lufthansa and Austrian Airlines (Gabel et al., 2011; Lufthansa, 2015). There are many benefits for the registered "Doctor on Board" passengers who become members under the Lufthansa Miles & More fly mile program. These include:

- ✈ 5,000 Miles & More award miles upon sign-up
- ✈ Up to 5,000 Miles & More award miles for each IFME assist
- ✈ Free Lufthansa's book "Handbook of Aviation Medicine and Inflight Medical Emergencies"
- ✈ A "Doctor on Board" luggage tag
- ✈ $50 Euros off the members next flight and future special promotions
- ✈ The opportunity to attend Lufthansa's German Academy for Aviation Medicine (2-day course)
- ✈ IFME liability insurance provided by Lufthansa German Airlines (Lufthansa, 2015)

In the event of an IFME aboard Lufthansa or Austrian Airlines, flight crews would be aware of the registered "Doctors on Board" and would contact them individually rather than alerting the entire cabin. Physicians under this program can register under one of six specialties, 1) anesthesiology, 2) general medicine, 3) internal medicine, 4) gynecology, 5) neurology/psychiatry, and 6) miscellaneous specialty (Gabel et al., 2011). Since credentials for the registered "Doctors on Board" have already been verified prior to the flight, the problem of physicians not having proper identification during an incident no longer exists. Currently, only physicians qualify for this program and they can register online at: http://www.lufthansa.com/us/en/Doctor-on-board.

1-3-2. TURKISH AIRLINES SMILING DOCTORS PROGRAM

A recent airline to implement a doctor on board program is Turkish Airline's, with their "Smiling Doctors" program. To become a member of the Turkish Airlines "Smiling Doctors" program, the passenger would first register as a member with the "Miles & Smiles" program and then apply for the "Smiling Doctors" program. The passenger benefits of a registered doctor include:

- 5,000 Bonus Miles after their first flight
- Registered Doctors will be given medical support from Turkish Airlines for IFMEs

(Turkish Airlines, 2017)

Physicians can register at: https://p.turkishairlines.com/en-us/miles-and-smiles/news/index.html

1-3-3. ANA DOCTORS ON BOARD SERVICE

In July of 2016, ANA Airlines began its "ANA Doctor On Board" service which states:

> "under the new service, should and injury, illness or other medical emergency occur midflight, cabin crew will no longer have to make an initial announcement...instead, they will be able to directly seek the help of any physicians on the flight who have registered in advance with the ANA Doctor On Board service, leading to a more rapid emergency response" (ANA Group, 2016, p. 1).

The main benefit of registering for the "ANA Doctors On Board" service according to ANA Airlines is that "under the new system, any injury or damage claims filed by passengers as a result medical treatment provided midflight will be handled by ANA," other than gross negligence by the doctor (ANA Group, 2016, p. 1). Licensed doctors can sign up for the "ANA Doctors On Board" service at: http://www.ana.co.jp/wws/us/e/wws_common/amc.

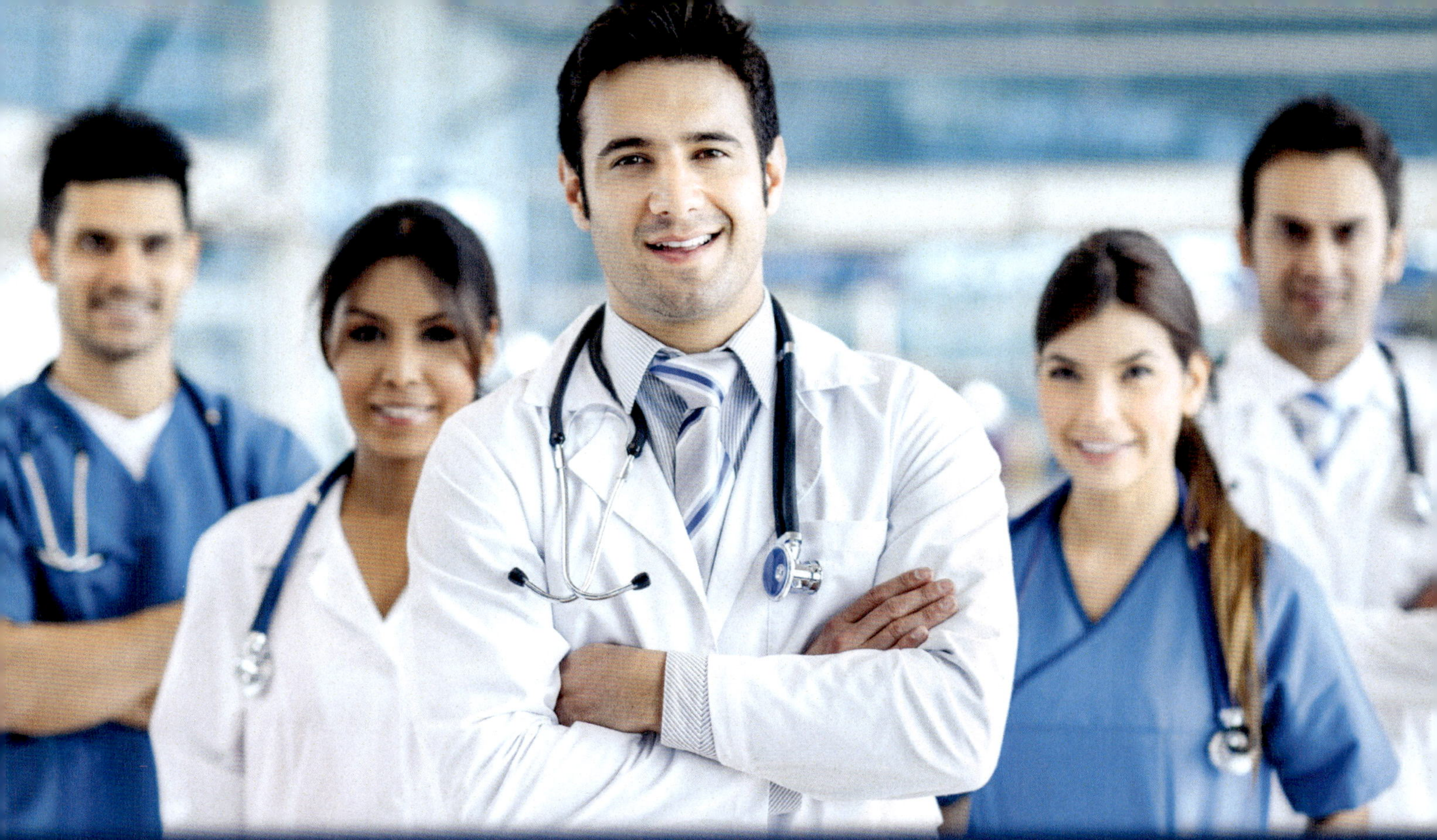

Chapter 2

MedLink and Ground-Based Airline Physicians

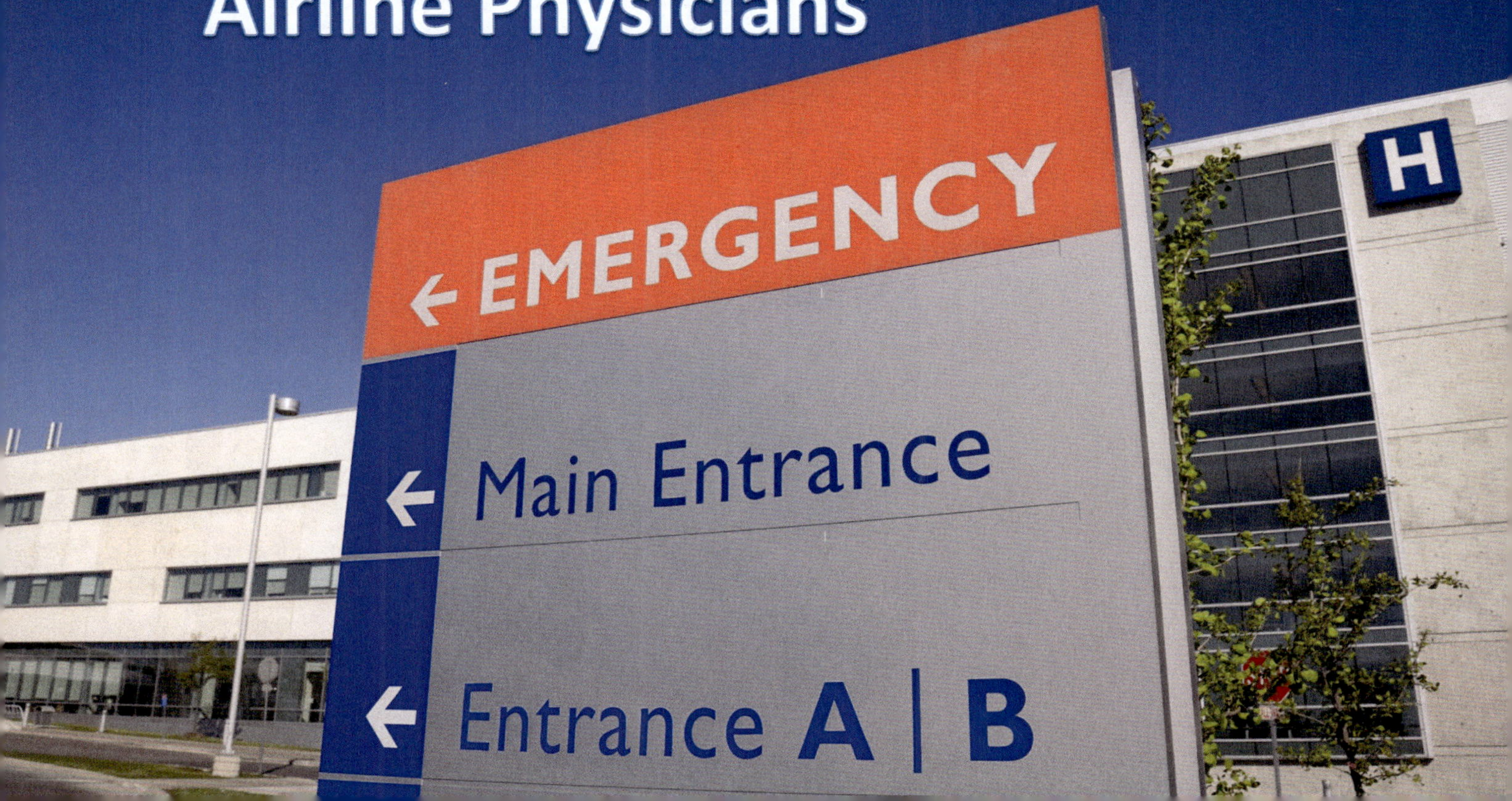

- ☑ Ground-Based Physicians Can Provide Medical Guidance to Off-Duty EMS Professionals
    - Administer Medication through Remote MedLink Physicians

✈ **How to Use the MedLink Service Worldwide (a MedAire Program)**

- ☑ MedLink Call Process
- ☑ Passenger Fit-to-Fly Assessments

✈ **Other Ground-Based Physician Services**

- ☑ Don't Be a Hero, Call MedLink First
- ☑ Diversion of Aircraft

✈ **MedLink Program Reduces the Risk of Potential Liability to Airlines and Crew**

✈ **MedAire website:** **http://www.medaire.com** (Alves, 2015; Harrison, 2006; MedAire, 2014)

2-1. U.S. COMMERCIAL AIRLINES HAVE ACCESS TO GROUND-BASED PHYSICIANS 24/7

Dr. Paulo Alves, the MedAire Global Medical Director, was interviewed regarding the company's aeronautical medical services including the MedLink program for aircraft. The MedLink program is described as an in-flight medical advisory service for airlines, both in the air and on the ground. When asked how many U.S. airlines utilize a ground-based physician service, Dr. Alves was certain that 100% of the U.S. airlines were either subscribers to the MedLink program or received ground-based physician services from another source. MedAire also provides training and medical equipment to over 60 airlines around the globe (Tobias, 2013).

The STAT-MD program, located at the University of Pittsburgh Medical Center, is a second provider for airline ground-based physician services. The STAT-MD program, which operates similarly to the MedLink program, is open 24 hours a day, and serves approximately 20 airlines worldwide (Tobias, 2013). A third ground-based physician service for airlines is a program called "The First Call." It is based in the ED at the Aberdeen Royal Infirmary in Scotland (The First Call, 2015).

Although the FAA and the EASA do not require airlines to have a ground-based physician program in place, most airlines worldwide and 100% inside the U.S. contract these services to MedLink, STAT-MD, The First Call, or through their own ground-based physician and/or medical advisory service. It is estimated that between MedLink and STAT-MD past call data, approximately 30,000 IFME calls are made by commercial airlines crews each year (Tobias, 2013; Peterson, et al., 2013).

Some countries such as France, provides airlines with no-cost medical advisory service's during an IFME over their territory, much like how the 911 system in the United States operates – but tailored for aircraft.

2-2. MAJORITY OF AIRLINES USE MEDAIRE'S MEDLINK SERVICE

MedAire, a leader in the international S.O.S. business, has become the majority stakeholder in providing airlines with the required medical equipment and related services. MedAire is the leader as the globe's 911 (remote area) emergency services provider when immediate medical help is not available. In fact, MedAire's MedLink service provides coverage to 115 airlines worldwide and is the largest provider of ground-based emergency physician services in the industry (MedAire, 2014). In addition to commercial aircraft, MedLink serves approximately 95% of the business aviation operators worldwide (MedAire, 2014).

2-2-1. INTRODUCTION ON MEDAIRE AND MEDLINK

MedAire was launched in 1986 by an ambitious entrepreneur named Joan McCorkle, she later changed her name to Joan Sullivan Garrett. After being unsuccessful in saving an 8-year old Arizona boy involved in an unintentional incident on a remote country road, Garrett had an unwavering vision to provide "the medical expertise of an emergency room at the scene of a remote medical emergency" (Harrison, 2006, p. 1). Her goal was to provide a system of advanced medical care when no such system was practical, such as when aboard commercial aircraft.

Garrett was no stranger to in-flight medical care, she had been a Samaritan Health flight nurse aboard medical response helicopters prior to creating MedAire and began her business by selling emergency medical kits (EMKs) to airlines (Harrison, 2006). The year 1986 was a great year for Garrett's new business, this happened to be the same year that the FAA mandated EMKs on all U.S. operated airlines. In late 1987, Garrett expanded MedAire's services to include "MedLink," a new service aimed at aircraft that incorporated remote emergency assistance through telemedicine methods and ground-based physicians. Today, Medaire's mission as an International SOS Company is to serve: 1) airline crews and passengers, 2) yacht crew and guests, and 3) business and general aviation.

2-2-2. MEDLINK'S REMOTE COMMUNICATIONS TO EMERGENCY ROOM PHYSICIANS

Banner Good Samaritan Hospital in Phoenix, Arizona, has a team of approximately 20 ED Physicians who work seven days a week, 24 hours a day answering incoming calls from airlines around the world urgently needing IFME consultations. Before a call is transferred to a MedLink physician, a call specialist initiates the call much like a 911 operator and determines if a translator is required. If a translator is required, MedLink has the ability to translate 140 different languages to ensure that no matter what language the airline crewmembers speak, they will receive the proper instructions to treat their ill passenger (MedAire, 2014). All MedLink physicians have specific knowledge and training regarding IFMEs which makes these medical professionals experts in dealing with IFMEs.

2-2-3. LACK OF MEDICAL PROFESSIONALS ON-BOARD

According to Dr. David Streitweiser, the MedLink Medical Director, there are many instances aboard airlines when there are no medical professionals available to help during an IFME and it can be difficult to get an accurate assessment of the patient's medical status (Brennan, 2013). This is the main reason for MedLink's service, even if an airplane was flying at 35,000 feet above the earth with no EMS services, MedLink physicians are available 24 hours a day, seven days a week (24/7) to help the crew or off-duty EMS professional with an IFME. Unfortunately, even though many of the United States based airlines subscribe to MedLink, they are slow to use the services (Alves, 2015). Therefore, more IFME training is needed within the airlines and EMS community.

2-2-4. GROUND PHYSICIANS CAN PROVIDE MEDICAL GUIDANCE TO OFF-DUTY EMS PROFESSIONALS

In the event of an IFME when an off-duty EMS professional is providing care alone, the rescuer should realize that he/she is not alone. The rescuer is just one call away from a MedLink or ground-based physician that can confirm or reject the on-board diagnosis and treatment plan. Additionally, in the event an off-duty EMS professional is not authorized to administer certain medications in his/her home state, when in-flight, there are exceptions to the rule. If the rescuer has been trained in the procedure and is a certified EMS professional, the rescuer would be allowed to administer those medications (e. g., Epi-Pen, I.V. fluids, nitroglycerin tablets) and be covered under the AMAA (regardless of state or local policies) and therefore be immune to state or federal liability while aboard an American registered aircraft. This holds true if the medical care rendered did not involve gross negligence or willful misconduct. "In summary, outside of gross negligence or willful misconduct, the AMAA protects from liability any physician (including nurse, paramedic, EMT) who renders emergency care even if that care is not rendered in the way that a reasonably medically qualified individual would have done so" (Stewart et al., 2013, p. 1776).

2-2-5. ADMINISTER MEDICATIONS THROUGH MEDLINK PHYSICIANS

The only airborne medical response to an IFME call for help would be from: 1) the flight attendants and 2) any volunteer off-duty EMS or medical professionals. Due to no immediate ground-based EMS options while in the air, an off-duty EMS professional may be called to help and asked to perform care not normally within their scope of certification.

Note: Always consult with a ground-based physician before providing any medications to patients.

If it is required to provide certain life-saving care or medications to an ill passenger in-flight with no other higher trained medical professional on-board, ground-based physicians shall make the call on treatment with the priority going to diversion of the aircraft to a close airport. If the only possible option for the patient's survival is the administration of certain medications outside the scope of the off-duty EMS professional's training, the ground-based doctor and/or the captain of the aircraft may have the authority to approve the treatment removing the liability from the off-duty EMS professional.

In 2010, Carol Glover, a registered nurse (RN) responded to an IFME on-board a commercial aircraft cruising at 30,000 feet and administered an I.V. to a dehydrated passenger without physician oversight. According to the editor's note in an article describing an IFME at 30,000 feet, "although starting an I.V. independent of a licensed prescriber isn't within the typical scope of an RN's practice, this action (as well as others) may be justified in certain life-threatening emergency situations, particularly when medical resources are lacking" (Glover, 2010, p. 45). This same principal would apply to off-duty EMS professionals if the actions appear necessary to save a life and no other medical resources are immediately available.

Note: It is recommended that after such an incident regarding an IFME, the off-duty EMS professional should ask the Captain for a signed letter offering immunity from liability.

2-3. HOW TO USE THE MEDLINK SERVICE WORLDWIDE (A MEDAIRE PROGRAM)

During an IFME that you have been summoned to by the crew, ensure that the MedLink in-flight medical advisory service or the appropriate ground-based physician has been contacted. Follow the recommended steps below when contacting MedLink (Campbell, 2007):

1. Ensure the scene is safe around the patient
2. Identify yourself to the patient and confirm consent or implied consent (for unconscious patient)
3. Perform preliminary assessment of the patient's condition and the seriousness of the emergency
4. Check ABCs, initiate CPR and/or AED use, if indicated
5. Request EMK or EEMK, O_2, AED as needed
6. Notify flight crews of the medical severity and request the MedLink Patch Checklist

List Continued on Next Page

7. Record patient data pertaining to the medical emergency on the MedLink Patch Checklist if available, you may request assistance from a flight crew member or volunteer to record the data. A generic airline patch checklist form is shown below:

Airline In-Flight Medical Advisory Checklist

	Patient / Medical Checklist - Check Each Line (Medical Info for Ground Based Physician)		Initiate Phone/Radio Patch with MedLink / STAT-MD (Provide Flight Info to Ground Based Physician)
	Incident / Flight # ______		1) Aircraft Registration Number: ______
	Crewmembers: ______		2) Aircraft Model (Type): ______
	Patient: ______		3) Origination, Destination: ______
	Age: ______ Gender: ______		4) Destination - Zulu ETA: ______
	Conscious (Y/N): ______		5) ⇦ Patient Information – Read from Other Side
	Oriented X (Time, Place, Ect.): ______		6) Patient Status: ______
	Chief Complaint: ______		7) Patient Treatment Area: ______
	B/P: ____/____ Pulse: ______ Resp: ______		8) Revised Destination ______
	Medical Alert Tag: ______		9) Revised Destination Zulu ETA: ______
	Medical History: ______ ______		10) Medical Assistance Needed (Y/N): ______ Assistance Upon Arrival: (Y/N): ______
	Current Meds: ______ ______		11) Notes: ______ ______
	Allergies: ______		

8. Indicate if suspected of an infectious disease – travel history
9. Ask crew to initiate satellite phone or air-to-ground communications (note: smaller planes generally do not have a phone available to the off-duty EMS professional and the pilots will initiate the patch)
10. MedLink Direct Phone from landline/satellite/cellular: **1-602-239-3627**
11. MedLink coordinators have the capability to translate more than 140 languages
12. If available, request air-to-ground satellite phone to communicate with the ground-based physician (Campbell, 2007; Stocke, 2015; MedAire, 2014).

2-3-1. MEDLINK CALL PROCESS

When the flight crew contacts the MedLink service, it would generally be initiated from the cockpit by either the Captain or the 1st Officer. In smaller commuter type aircraft, generally the only method of communicating with MedLink will be the air-to-ground radio system located in the cockpit; in larger aircraft, there may be additional communication systems including satellite telephones and/or crew intercom phones that may be patched with MedLink (Stocke, 2015).

Once the MedLink call specialist receives the IFME call from the flight crew, the MedLink call coordinator will coordinate the entire call, gather pertinent information from the completed MedLink Patch Checklist, and then immediately refer the caller to the appropriate MedLink physician located at the Banner Good Samaritan Hospital in Phoenix, Arizona (Campbell, 2007; Harrison, 2006). MedAire provides a one-stop solution for complete IFME care from EMK equipment to ground-based physicians, so you can be assured that the MedLink referred physician will be trained in IFME procedures including the EMK contents on each particular airline. In instances where an off-duty EMS professional is not aware of specific medical equipment available to them during the IFME, the MedLink physician will advise the off-duty EMS professional and/or the crew regarding the emergency equipment available on-board (Campbell, 2007).

MedLink is also available to the flight crew and off-duty EMS professionals (by landline/satellite/cellular phone; **1-602-239-3627**) while on the ground at an airport, terminal gate, on a taxiway/runway, or for emergency purposes if the aircraft has crashed or landed in a remote location. There may be situations that an IFME has resulted from an unforeseen in-flight related emergency resulting in the plane landing in an area far from rescue personnel or immediate medical care. In this situation, MedAire would be able to assist with the treatment of patients on the ground prior to rescue personnel arriving.

2-3-2. PASSENGER FIT-TO-FLY ASSESSMENTS

When questions arise at the airport regarding the possibility of an infirmed passenger, the affected airline is encouraged to call MedAire for a fit-to-fly medical assessment of that passenger prior to boarding the flight

(MedAire, 2014). By conducting a MedAire fit-to-fly assessment over the phone with a MedLink physician prior to flight, airlines can prevent a possible IFME from occurring altogether. Persons who may be suffering from certain respiratory/cardiovascular illnesses and/or diseases may be unaware that air travel may worsen their symptoms while in-flight.

2-4. OTHER GROUND-BASED PHYSICIAN SERVICES

Not all airlines use MedAire EMKs and/or contract for the MedLink service. If an airline uses an internal airline physician, the steps for contacting the airline physician would be similar to the MedLink process as shown below:

1. Ensure you have been summoned to help by flight crew
2. Ensure the scene is safe around the patient
3. Perform preliminary assessment of the patient's condition and the seriousness of the emergency
4. Identify yourself to the patient and confirm consent or implied consent (for unconscious patient)
5. Check ABCs, initiate CPR and/or AED use if indicated
6. Request EMK or EEMK, O_2, AED as needed
7. Notify flight crews of the medical severity and request the airline ground-based physician checklist
8. Record patient data pertaining to the medical emergency
9. Indicate if suspected of an infectious disease – travel history
10. Ask crew to initiate satellite phone or air-to-ground communications
11. If available, request air-to-ground satellite phone to communicate with the ground-based physician (Campbell, 2007; Stocke, 2015).

2-4-1. DON'T BE A HERO, CALL MEDLINK FIRST

Dr. Alves, the MedAire Global Medical Director stated in an interview the importance related to IFMEs was to not make the situation worse in-flight. Medical treatment inside a passenger aircraft is cramped, dark, loud, and impractical in terms of privacy and comfort. When involved in an IFME, it is always the best practice to stabilize the patient with the least invasive treatments possible. "Don't try to be a Hero," keep the treatment simple, and have the flight crew contact MedLink immediately when an IFME is apparent (Alves, 2015).

Unfortunately, this does not always happen. Dr. Alves has been made aware of situations where volunteer physicians have worsened the medical condition of a patient in-flight, which could have been avoided if a ground-based physician trained in IFMEs was contacted prior to treatment. Current IFME data on types of medical symptoms occurring in-flight are overwhelmingly categorized as non-life threatening and the majority of people ill in-flight do not need to be transported or admitted to a hospital (Chandra & Conry, 2013; Silverman & Gendreau, 2008). Deaths in-flight are extremely rare and in all the IFME studies reviewed, death occurrences were reported to be as low as 0.3% to 1.3% when reflected in the overall medical incidents studied (Peterson et al., 2013).

2-4-2. DIVERSION OF AIRCRAFT

If the ground-based physician determines that a diversion of the aircraft is warranted due to the IFME, the captain would be informed with pertinent information where he or she could make the ultimate decision to divert the flight to a closer airport (Campbell, 2007). The captain of the airplane has the final say in whether to divert or to continue on to the final destination. Certain medical emergencies have a higher occurrence of diversions, especially on international flights. These IFMEs would include:

- ✓ Cardiac 26.4% (chest pain most common)
- ✓ Neurological 19.5% (stroke most common)
- ✓ Gastrointestinal 11.4%
- ✓ Syncope 10% (Rahim Valani, 2010)

Note: For more information on diversions, refer to: Chapter 9: Highlights – Diversion of Aircraft.

Chapter Notes

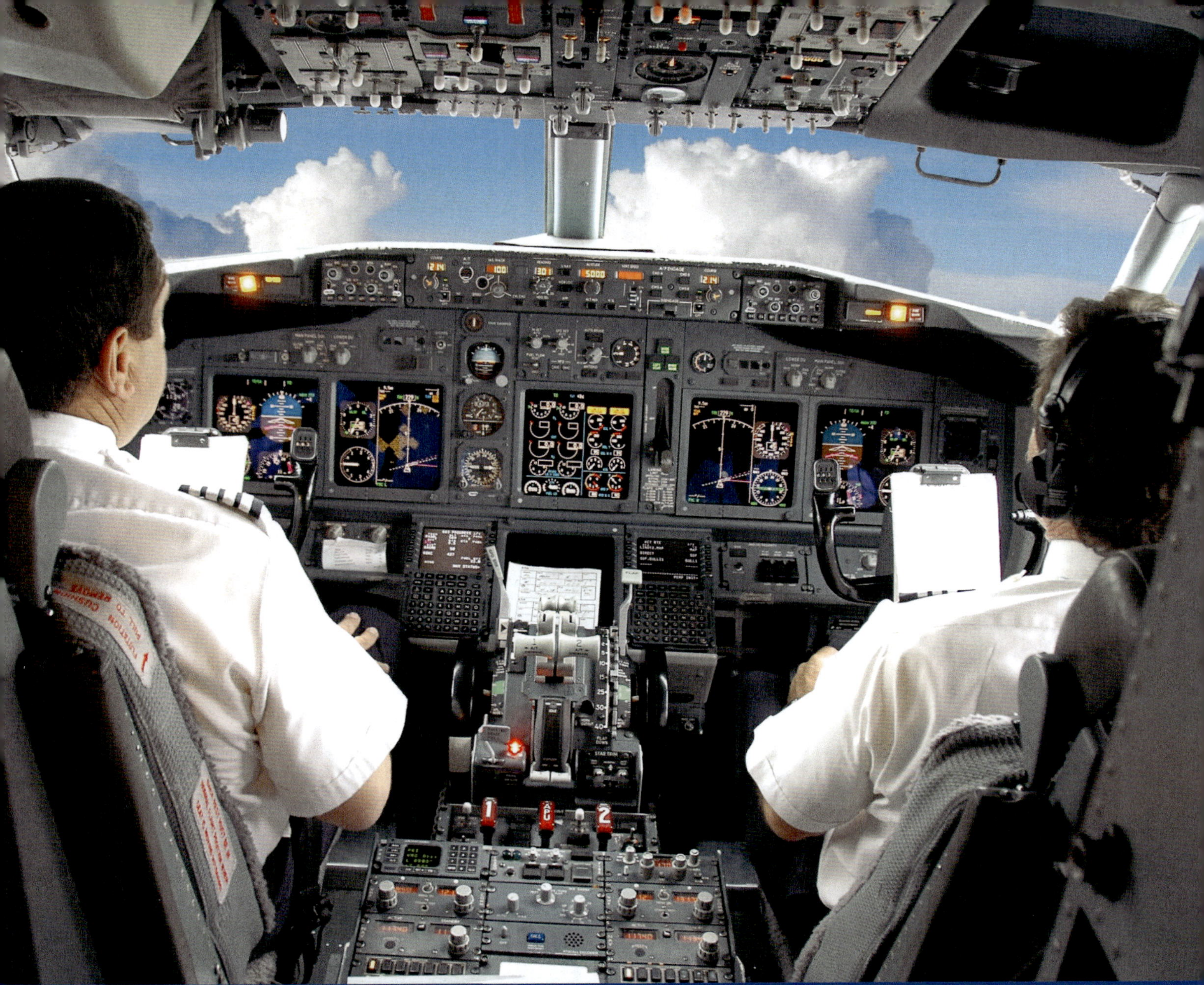

Chapter 3

The Captain, Crew and Passengers

CHAPTER 3: HIGHLIGHTS - THE CAPTAIN OF THE PLANE AND FLIGHT CREW

- **Captain is the "King of the Castle"**
  - ☑ Captain Can Approve/Deny Medical Treatment by Volunteers On-Board
  - ☑ Captain Can Over-Ride the Recommendations of a Physician or Medical Professional
  - ☑ Captain Has the Final Say Related to Conflicts on the Plane
- **Pilots Positions and Duties in the Cockpit**
  - ☑ Captain
  - ☑ 1st Officer
  - ☑ Pilots Responsible for The Safe Fight of The Aircraft
    - Pilots fly the plane
  - ☑ Cockpit is a Secure Location with an Armored Door
- **Crewmember's Duties in the Back of the Aircraft**
  - ☑ Flight Attendants
    - Responsible for the passenger compartment of the aircraft
    - Respond to emergencies in the passenger compartment
    - Unlocking the Lavatory from the Outside
    - Hidden Crew Rest Areas
- **Pilots Request Ground-Based Physician Assistance**
  - ☑ Pilots Assist with MedLink or Ground-Based Physician Assistance
  - ☑ Flight Attendants Coordinate Medical Treatment with the Passengers
- **Three types of passengers and their medical conditions**
  - ☑ Unknown Conditions
  - ☑ Predisposed Conditions
  - ☑ Known Conditions

3-1. CAPTAIN – KING OF THE CASTLE

Physicians may be accustomed to having their orders followed when working in their own medical facilities. Some medical professionals may believe they are the "king of the castle" when working at their own clinical practice, this may be true on the ground but it is not the case when in-flight on commercial aircraft (Gabel et al., 2011, p. 47). It is important to remember that the Captain of the aircraft is technically the "king of the castle" while in-flight and has the highest authority on the plane (Gabel et al., 2011). According to the German Aviation Safety Law known as "Luftsicherheitsgesetz", the Captain of an aircraft has the equivalent enforcement powers of a policeman (Graf et al., 2012).

3-1-1. CAPTAIN CAN APPROVE/DENY MEDICAL TREATMENT BY VOLUNTEERS

IFMEs tend to occur at the worst possible times and to make matters worse, there are many occasions when no medically trained professionals are available to assist. This puts the safety of all on-board at risk, especially when passengers are demanding help from the flight crew. In situations like this, flight crews rely heavily on the expertise of the medical staff at MedLink. When no medially trained personnel are on-board, it is possible for MedLink physicians with authorization from the captain, to approve specific medical interventions through passengers who are willing to help. One such example can be demonstrated when a passenger is suddenly stricken with life-threatening anaphylactic shock from a food allergy, causing the patient to have respiratory distress and become unresponsive. MedLink physicians would most likely recommend the immediate administration of epinephrine through an EpiPen auto-injector located in the EEMK. In such a case, which would be classified as an extreme emergency, the captain in consultation with a MedLink physician may choose to authorize a non-medically trained passenger to administer the EpiPen while being instructed by a MedLink physician. Although scenarios like the one above are rare, when the only alternative to treatment is certain death, the captain of the aircraft does have authority to approve medical treatment that would otherwise be unavailable in-flight.

The captain of the aircraft also has the authority to deny a passenger the right to attend to another ill passenger. Situations where this may occur is when an off-duty EMS professional or physician offers to help during an IFME but does not have proof of medical qualifications or the volunteer medical professional appears to be under the influence of a substance. In this situation, the captain would be able to either approve the assistance by the volunteer or confirm the flight crew's refusal. Once the captain makes a decision, that decision is final.

3-1-2. CAPTAIN CAN OVERRULE THE RECOMMENDATIONS OF A MEDICAL PROFESSIONAL

To ensure the safe travel of all on-board, the captain of an aircraft may over-ride the medical related recommendations of an off-duty EMS professional or other medically trained professional. The captain is the best suited person on an aircraft to determine the safest plan for obtaining ground-based medical assistance for an ill passenger. When flying over an ocean, it is quite clear that there are few viable options other than turning back or diverting to the nearest airport. The captain and/or the flight crew will most likely contact MedLink or similar service for consultation with ground-based physicians on what options are available. In many instances, the captain will rely more heavily on the recommendations from a MedLink physician rather than the volunteer medical professional, even if the chosen decision is not best for the patient. There are additional risks and dangers related to diversion of an aircraft, especially if the intended airport is unknown to the captain.

The captain of an aircraft shall comply with all laws pertaining to the aircraft's particular jurisdiction. Within the EASAs jurisdiction for example, the captain shall ensure adherence to certain laws related to IFMEs. JAA regulations (JAR-OPS 1.775) mandates that the aircraft Captain "shall ensure that drugs are not administered other than by qualified doctors, nurses, or similarly qualified personnel" (Cocks & Liew, 2007, p. 4). Violations of this regulation and others can result in the arrest of the captain, the entire flight crew, and the medical professional(s) attending to the IFME.

In 1999, Dr. Tamas Major, along with the entire flight crew on-board a Hungarian National Airlines flight, were arrested by Turkish authorities upon landing when it was discovered that their combative IFME patient had died after being injected with 10 mg of diazepam (Kovac, 1999). Passengers reported that this combative and delusional man was attacking people including the captain and had attempted to light a female's hair on fire with a lighter (Kovac). It was later determined that the passenger was under an alcohol/drug induced psychosis and had possibly died as a result of his violent behavior and drug intoxication. All arrested, (including the captain) because of this incident, were released shortly after their arrest by Turkish authorities pending autopsy results (Kovac, 1999). This incident is a sobering reminder that when patients die during IFMEs, everyone involved could be arrested upon landing in a foreign nation. Due to the lack of follow-up articles on this incident, it appears that no criminal charges were ever filed against Dr. Major or the flight crew.

3-1-3. CONFLICTS IN-FLIGHT – CAPTAIN HAS THE FINAL SAY

When there is a conflict between the flight crew and an off-duty EMS professional, the captain of the aircraft will have the final say, regardless if the decision results in a negative outcome. The captain's primary objective is to safely fly the aircraft from point A to B, while the crewmember's primary objective is to care for and manage the passenger compartment during the flight (Stocke, 2015).

3-2. PILOTS POSITIONS AND DUTIES IN THE COCKPIT

In general, the flight crew consists of the pilots (i.e., Captain and 1st Officer) and one or more flight attendants, depending on the size of the aircraft. Transcontinental aircraft may carry additional crewmembers in the cockpit such as relief pilots/crews due to the extended time in-flight.

3-2-1. CAPTAIN AND 1ST OFFICER

The crew located on the flight deck includes the Captain and 1st Officer; these pilots have the primary responsibility for the safe flying of the aircraft (Stocke, 2015). The captain's seat is always on the left side of the cockpit and the 1st Officer's is always on the right side. Cockpits are generally very cramped on smaller aircraft and quite large on long-haul aircraft. After the terrorist attacks on 911, airlines around the world have fortified cockpit doors with extensive armor reinforcement that offers protection against unauthorized access and both bullet/explosive protection. Due to these security measures, passengers are not allowed inside the cockpit unless they are requested in an emergency. Air France released a study over a 20-year period demonstrating that of their 1800 pilots, a total of 10 pilots had suffered a medical emergency in the cockpit which incapacitated them and required assistance from the flight crew and passengers (Rushkin, Hernandez, & Barash, 2008).

3-3. CREWMEMBERS DUTIES IN THE REAR OF THE AIRCRAFT

While it is the flight crew's duty to safely fly the aircraft from the cockpit, it is the flight attendant's duty to manage the rear of the aircraft. Commercial aircraft are generally custom built according to each airline's specifications, some include crew rest areas, cargo areas, patient transport compartments, and emergency equipment compartments.

3-3-1. HIDDEN CREW REST AREAS

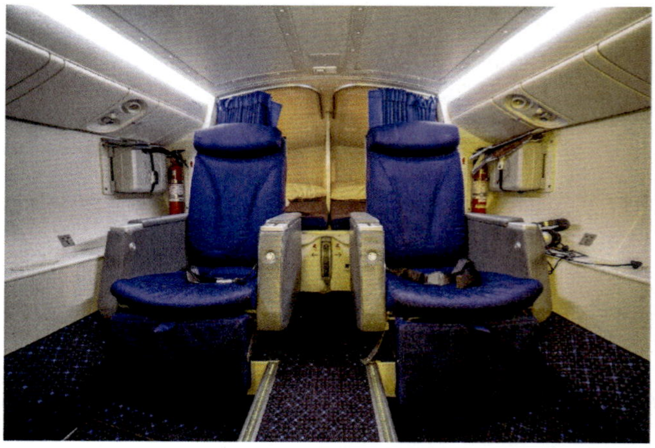
Hidden Crew Rest Area Available on Wide-Body Aircraft

Many modern 747, 777, 787 and other long-haul commercial aircraft are equipped with crew rest areas inside the cabin. Generally, these rest areas are built above the passenger compartment and are only accessible to the crew. The crew rest area pictured to the right includes two comfortable seats, and located behind the seats, are two comfortable beds. New Boeing 777-300ER aircraft can be ordered with a crew rest area of up to 10-bunk beds which can be accessed through the rear of the plane. The crew rest area is accessible through a hidden stairway. The stairway leads to the top of the cabin, above the passenger compartment. The crew rest area is located in the celling directly over the passenger compartment – hidden from view!

3-3-2. FLIGHT ATTENDANTS

The flight attendant's primary objective is to ensure the safety of the passengers within the passenger compartment of the aircraft. The flight attendants run the operation of caring for the passengers while the pilots safely fly the plane. It is extremely rare for a pilot to walk through the passenger compartment in-flight; this would be generally done during an emergency where an inspection of the aircraft is needed.

When an emergency does present itself in-flight, the flight attendants "can't call 911, they are 911" (Davis & DeBarros, 2008, p. 3). Flight attendants are well trained in airline safety and are staffed on flights to ensure the safety of all the passengers on-board. Flight attendants are trained in basic first aid/CPR and will communicate the IFME to the flight deck and other crewmembers during an emergency to facilitate a course of action. In the case of an IFME, flight attendants rely heavily on off-duty EMS professionals for proper medical care.

3-3-3. CABIN CHIMES – EMERGENCY CREWMEMBER COMMUNICATIONS

In the event of an IFME, retired American Airline crewmember Shawn Lynn noted "that the crew is alerted to a medical emergency by four rings of the planes aircrafts chime" (Davis & DeBarros, 2008, p. 3). Other airlines may use four rings of the chime for a general emergency or other urgent matter. This procedure of notifying the crew may differ for each airline, but it shall be noted that the airline industry does heavily use the chime system in-flight on a regular basis.

3-3-4. EMERGENCY IN THE LAVATORY – HOW TO UNLOCK THE DOOR FROM THE OUTSIDE

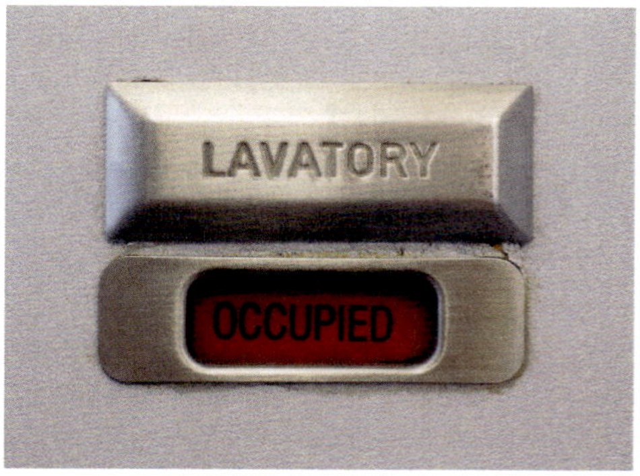

Commercial aircraft lavatories are small and cramped, if an IFME occurred inside one and the patient was unable to unlock the door, how would a flight attendant or first responder unlock the door? Airline manufactures have already solved this problem by allowing lavatory doors to be locked and unlock from the outside. "On some aircraft, unlocking the door is as simple as lifting up the 'lavatory' sign and sliding over the toggle switch located underneath the cover" (Zhang, 2016, p. 4). Airline manufactures may utilize different locations and/or systems for lavatory door lock mechanisms, always ask a flight attendant for assistance when attempting to unlock a lavatory door from the outside.

3-3-5. FIGHT ATTENDANT AND PILOTS WORK TOGETHER TO CONTACT GROUND-BASED PHYSICIANS

When it is determined by an off-duty EMS professional or by a flight attendant that a ground-based physician must be contacted for an IFME, there is no standardized method of contacting the ground-based physician. Once the captain is notified of the request for the MedLink physician or similar service, the captain or first officer will begin the procedure for establishing an open communication portal with MedLink. In smaller commuter type aircraft, generally the only method of communicating with MedLink will be the air-to-ground radio system located in the cockpit in conjunction with flight checklists of aeronautical radio channels for different stations across the country (Stocke, 2015). The process of contacting a ground-based physician in smaller and older aircraft is not as easy as one may think. It is common for a radio/phone patch with a ground-based physician to take 5-15 minutes (or longer) to become established. Some locations in the world may require old technology high frequency radio waves to contact a ground-based physician. Over vast oceans, there may be areas where radio communication is non-existent. With the implementation of satellite phones, the process of contacting a MedLink physician is quicker and more accurate.

3-4. THREE TYPES OF PASSENGERS AND THEIR MEDICAL CONDITIONS

When categorizing types of passengers who experience an IFME event, there are three classifications:

- Unknown Conditions – Unexpected Medical Issue
- Predisposed Conditions – Underlying Medical Condition
- Known Conditions – Seeking Care Away from Home (Campbell, 2007).

Persons who have a known medical complication and/or disease will have additional difficulty breathing while in-flight due to the reduced partial pressure of O_2 in the cabin. MedAire or an airline ground-based physician service can be consulted regarding an ill passenger prior to departure to ensure the passenger is healthy enough to travel by air (by landline/satellite/cellular phone; **1-602-239-3627** Passenger Fit-to-Fly Assessments).

3-4-1. LUFTHANSA PATIENT TRANSPORT COMPARTMENT (PTC)

Lufthansa is the only airline in the world that offers a Patient Transport Compartment (PTC) service for the safe transportation of intensive care patients. Lufthansa created their PTC (pictured to the right) to replicate a medical facility and is designed much like an air ambulance except for the fact that the PTC is utilized on jumbo jets (Lufthansa Medical Service, 2012). The Lufthansa PTC service began in 1999 and is available on most long-haul 747-400, A330, and A340 aircraft (Lufthansa Group, 2015). Lufthansa claims that the advantages of the PTC over an air ambulance service is a 50% reduction in patient transportation time.

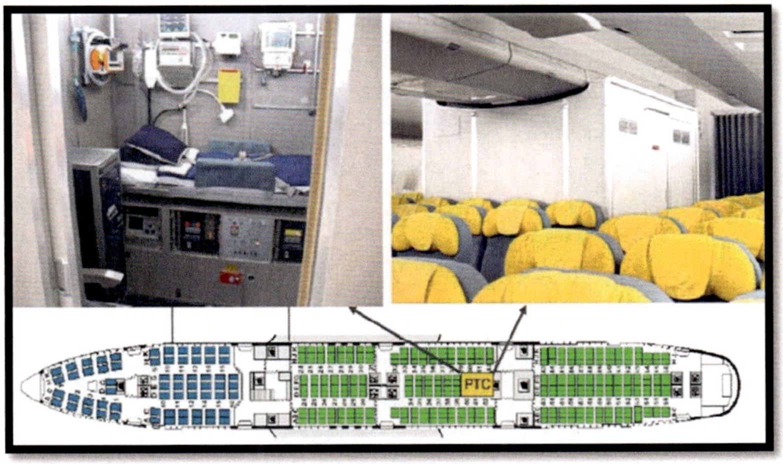

Lufthansa Patient Transport Compartment (PTC) on 747-400, A300, A340

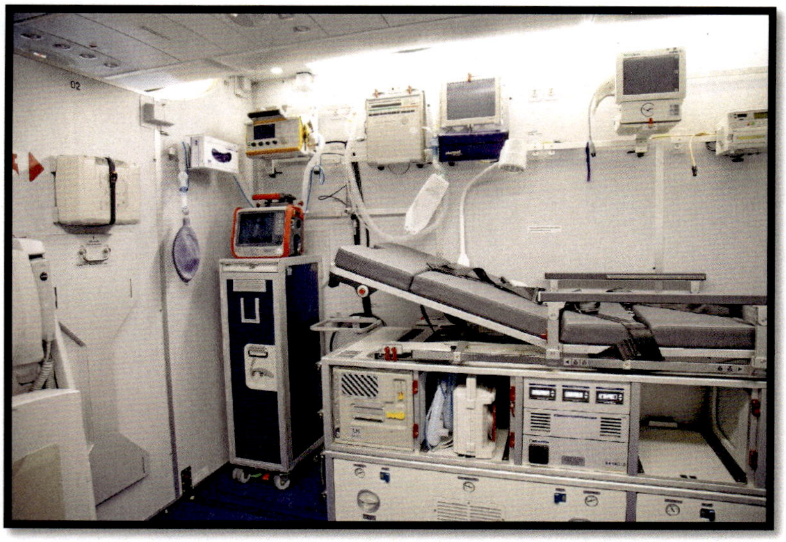
Lufthansa Patient Transport Unit Next Generation (PTU NG) on A380, 747-800

Lufthansa Airlines is upgrading their successful PTC service with a new product called the Patient Transport Unit Next Generation (PTU NG), this state-of-the-art medical transportation facility will be fitted on all newly acquired Airbus A380 and Boeing 747-800 aircraft (Lufthansa, n.d.).

Note: If responding to an IFME on-board a Lufthansa 747-400, 747-800, A330, A340, or A380 and the patient needs to be moved from their seat for immediate lifesaving medical treatment, ask a flight attendant if the PTC or the PTU NG is available. IF the PTC or PTU NG is not being utilized, ask for permission from the flight crew to use the onboard medical facility.

Chapter Notes

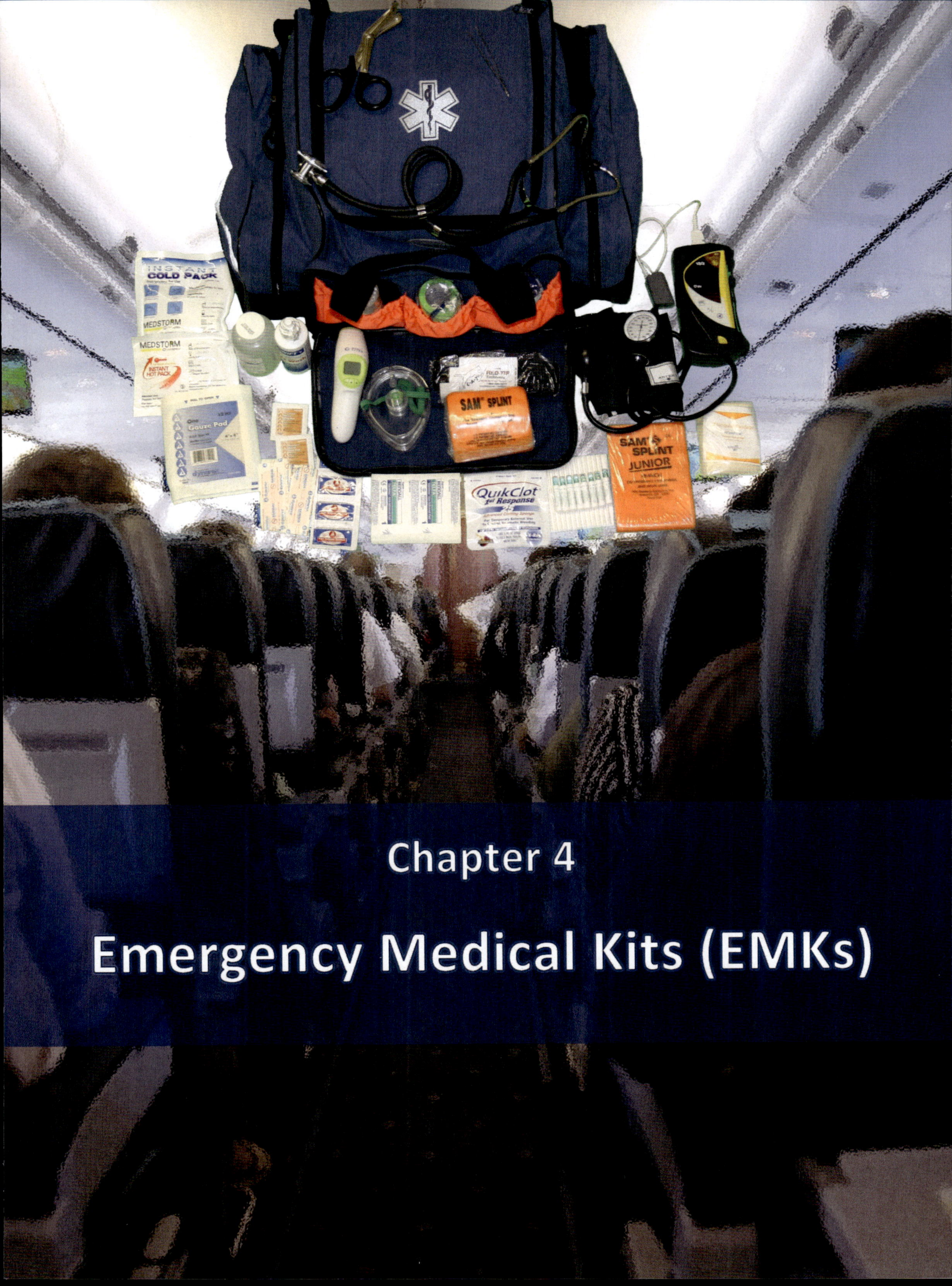

Chapter 4

Emergency Medical Kits (EMKs)

CHAPTER 4: HIGHLIGHTS – EMERGENCY MEDICAL KITS

- **Brief History of Aircraft Medical Kits**
  - ☑ Types of Aircraft Medical Kits
  - ☑ Difference between the AFAK, EMK, and EEMK
  - ☑ European Union (EU) Airlines May Call their EMK a First Aid Kit
    - (EU) Cabin Attendant Medical Kit (CAMK) – Similar to FAK
    - (EU) Doctors Kit – Similar to the EEMK
- **Contents of Aircraft Medical Kits**
  - ☑ Minimum Medical Components Required by the FAA/EASA
  - ☑ First Aid Kit (FAK) and Aircraft First Aid Kit (AFAK)
    - Designed for Flight Crew and First-Aid Volunteers
    - Required by the FAA/EASA for Commercial Airlines
  - ☑ Emergency Medical Kit (EMK)
    - Required by the FAA/EASA for Commercial Airlines
  - ☑ Enhanced Emergency Medical Kit (EEMK)
    - MedAire's EMK "Enhanced" for the Commercial Airline Industry
  - ☑ Doctor's Kit
    - Lufthansa Exclusive – Designed for Physicians with a Greater Selection of Medications and Airways
  - ☑ Optional Add-On Kits
    - Telemedicine Unit
    - Pediatrician Kit
    - Universal Precaution Kit (UPK)
- **Persons Allowed to use Medical Kits**

4-1. HISTORY OF FAA REGULATIONS REGARDING MEDICAL KITS

Beginning in 1986, the FAA has mandated that commercial aircraft operating in the United States (including international flights to and from the United States) incorporate Emergency Medical Kits (EMKs) in addition to First Aid Kits (FAKs) that were already in service on commercial airline fleets (Hordinsky & George, 1991). The implementation of EMKs on-board commercial aircraft has been regularly reviewed since the early 1980s with several medical equipment improvements. These improvements over the years have included:

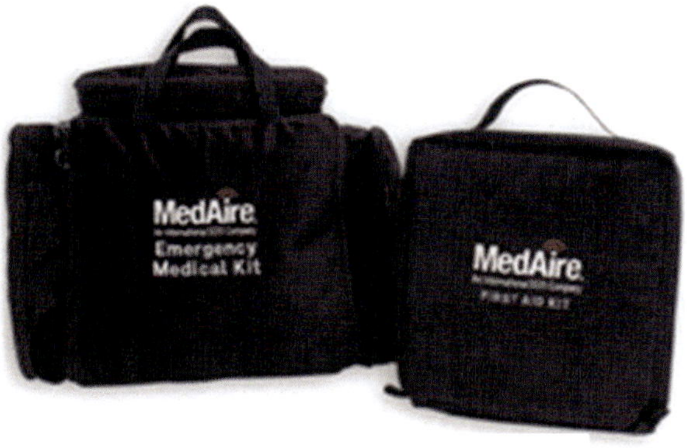

MedAire, EMK & FAK

- 1986 – FAA mandated EMK on Commercial Airlines
- 1994 – Add Protective Gloves to EMKs
- 1995 – EMKs Extended to Commuter Flights with One Flight Attendant
- 1998 – Added AEDs Requirement for Airlines
- 1998 – Added Good Samaritan Provision
- 2002 – Medication Upgrades to EMKs
- 2006 – Crewmember Training for AED use and Enhanced EMK Contents

(Federal Aviation Administration, 2006; Sirven, 2006)

4-2. TYPES OF AIRCRAFT MEDICAL KITS

- Passenger Service Kit (PSK)
- First Aid Kit (FAK) & Aircraft First Aid Kit (AFAK)
- Emergency Medical Kit (EMK) & Enhanced Emergency Medical Kit (EEMK)
- Doctor's Kit
- Pediatrician Kit
- Passenger Restraint Kit
- Universal Precaution Kit (UPK)
- Obstetrical Kit (MedAire, 2014)

Note: Many airlines will first offer the FAK or AFAK to off-duty EMS professionals; before the FAK or AFAK is opened, request the EMK or EEMK (Silverman & Gendreau, 2008). **Some airlines may place tamper seals on their medical kits to ensure they have not been tampered with prior to use** (Stocke, 2015).

4-2-1. DIFFERENCE BETWEEN THE TYPES OF AIRCRAFT MEDICAL KITS

There are several kits on-board commercial aircraft that may be available to the off-duty EMS professional depending on each airline's preference and the qualifications of each individual volunteer. Many aircraft medical kits are sealed by the airlines with tamper-proof devices for security and to ensure contents have not been tampered with. The contents in most of these kits are considered "No-Go" items and if used in flight, must be replaced/restocked when the flight has landed (Stocke, 2015). The only exception to this policy is with the PSK which is designed for simple first aid items (i.e. providing a bandage). MedAire's medical kits generally include a contents list and the location of those items.

Note: Medical suppliers such as MedAire design slightly different FAKs/EMKs for commercial airline and business aviation customers. Examples of both types of FAKs/EMKs are included in this manual.

4-2-2. PASSENGER SERVICE KIT (PSK)

The PSK is a very basic mini first aid kit with bandages, aspirin, Tylenol, antacid, and other minor simple/common-need items that can be handed out by the flight crew without opening a sealed, more advanced medical kit (MedAire, 2014). The PSK is not an item that is mandated by regulation and no medical training is required to use the medical supplies within the kit.

4-2-3. FIRST AID KIT (FAK) & AIRCRAFT FIRST AID KIT (AFAK)

The standard first-aid kit on-board commercial airlines may be the called the first aid kit (FAK) or aircraft first aid kit (AFAK). The FAK/AFAK are both designed to be used by the flight crew and non-medically trained professionals. The FAK/AFAK contains many items in a standard first aid kit such as gloves, bandages, cold packs, and additional medical items found in a standard kit. The AFAK contains additional basic life support equipment such as a stethoscope and blood pressure cuff, CPR mask, and various tablet medicines such as aspirin (Campbell, 2007). The FAK and the AFAK both meet requirements for the Code of Federal Regulations 121.803(c) (1), approved first aid kits (MedAire, 2014). It shall be noted that there is a minimum number of first aid kits required according to the number of passengers on a commercial aircraft as indicated in table 3 below:

4-2-4. FIRST AID-KITS REQUIRED PER PASSENGER COUNT

No. of passenger seats	No. of first-aid kits
0-50	1
51-150	2
151-250	3
More than 250	4

Table 3, Minimum Number of FAK per Passenger Seat, Source: U.S. Government Publishing Office, 2015d

4-2-5. EMERGENCY MEDICAL KIT (EMK) & ENHANCED EMERGENCY MEDICAL KIT (EEMK)

The next level of medical kit on-board aircraft is called the EMK and is generally reserved for off-duty EMS professionals and other medical professionals. The FAA requires EMKs on all commercial aircraft that can carry a payload of more than 7500 pounds (30 or more seats) and that has at least one flight attendant (Federal Aviation Administration, 2006). Since general aviation and certain charter aircraft carry EMKs in addition to commercial airlines, MedAire has named its EMK designed specifically for the airline industry as the Enhanced Emergency Medical Kit (EEMK). Both the EMK and the EEMK have all the FAA mandated medical components with the option of customization including additional components for each airline's needs. It is important for each off-duty EMS professional to consult with each individual airline for the kits it may carry on-board its aircraft.

To clarify the difference between the EMK and the EEMK, these two kits are essentially the same per FAA and EASA regulations. MedAire, a medical equipment provider of both the EMK and EEMK products, markets the EMK primarily for civilian/corporate aircraft while the EEMK is designed specifically for the commercial airline industry (Campbell, 2007). Most of the enhanced medical kits on-board commercial aircraft will be called the EEMK (Stocke, 2015). The FAA uses the EMK language within their regulations to describe the minimum components airlines are required to carry in their medical kits, but this does not mean airlines must use an EMK per se, just as long as their kits include the FAA/EASA minimum components. The EMK and the EEMK both meet requirements for the Code of Federal Regulations 121.803(c) (3), approved EMKs effective as of April 12, 2004 (MedAire, 2014; U.S. Government Publishing Office, 2015c).

4-2-6. DOCTORS KIT

Some international airlines such as Lufthansa Airlines also carry in addition to the EEMK, a "doctor's kit" which stores additional medical supplies and/or medications; these kits are generally reserved specifically for physicians for the treatment of life-threatening conditions (Gabel et al., 2011). The Doctors Kits will contain more advanced medical equipment such as endotracheal tubes/laryngoscope and additional medications.

4-2-7. PEDIATRICIAN KIT

The pediatrician kit may or may not be available on the specific airline flight in question. This kit is optional and is primarily reserved for families with children. The contents of this kit are designed specifically for treating pediatric illnesses.

4-2-8. PASSENGER RESTRAINT KIT

There are situations when a passenger may become unruly and/or agitated for unknown reasons and may even become combative with the cabin crew or other passengers. This presents a significant danger and threat in-flight to the other passengers, the crew, and the aircraft. To safely control the combative passenger without the use of sedatives, MedAire manufactures a passenger restraint kit. If a situation arises where a passenger needs to be detained and/or restrained for either his/her safety or the safety of everyone else on-board, immediately request the passenger restraint kit from the flight crew.

4-2-9. EUROPEAN UNION (EU) AIRLINES MAY CALL THEIR MEDICAL KITS DIFFERENT NAMES

Although essentially the same in terms of contents and medications, the airlines within the European Union (EU) may call their medical kits different names. The EU kits are generally called:

1. EU "Cabin Attendant Medical Kit" (CAMK) – Similar to the U.S. FAK
2. EU "First Aid Kit" (FAK) – Similar to the U.S. EMK
3. EU "Emergency Medical Kit" (EMK) – Same as U.S. EMK
4. EU "Doctors Kit" – Similar to the U.S. EEMK (Gabel, et al., 2011)

Note: The Doctors Kit does contain a much larger selection of medical drugs including Morphine and Diazepam. Some airlines have chosen to no longer carry Diazepam because it's a highly-restricted drug.

4-3. REQUIRED CONTENTS - AIRCRAFT MEDICAL KITS

Both the United States and the European Union (EU) require that all airlines conducting air travel to or from these countries, comply with their respective FAA and ESAS regulations. Many other countries that are not part of the European Union must still comply with these regulations if they want to conduct air travel within the United States or EU. For this reason, FAK and EMK manufactures base their standard kit packages on both the FAA and the EASA regulations. If EASA regulations dictate a requirement for additional medical supplies on EU based EMK's (when compared to FAA regulations), the U.S. based airlines' that operate in the EU shall meet these same EASA regulations. Represented in the following two tables are the minimum FAK and EMK contents based on FAA regulations. Table 4 (below) represents the FAA required contents for the FAK or the AFAK and Table 5 (page 53) represents the FAA required contents for the EMK or the EEMK.

4-3-1. FAA REQUIRED FAK OR AFAK CONTENTS (1 – 4 PER AIRCRAFT SIZE)

FAK Contents	Quantity
Adhesive bandage compresses, 1-inch	16
Antiseptic swabs	20
Ammonia inhalants	10
Bandage compresses, 4-inch	8
Triangular bandage compresses, 40-inch	5
Arm splint, non-inflatable	1
Leg splint, non-inflatable	1
Roller bandage, 4-inch	4
Adhesive tape, 1-inch standard roll	2
Bandage scissors	1

Table 4, FAA Required FAK Contents, Source: U.S. Government Publishing Office, 2015d

An Airbus A380 Requires (4) FAKs

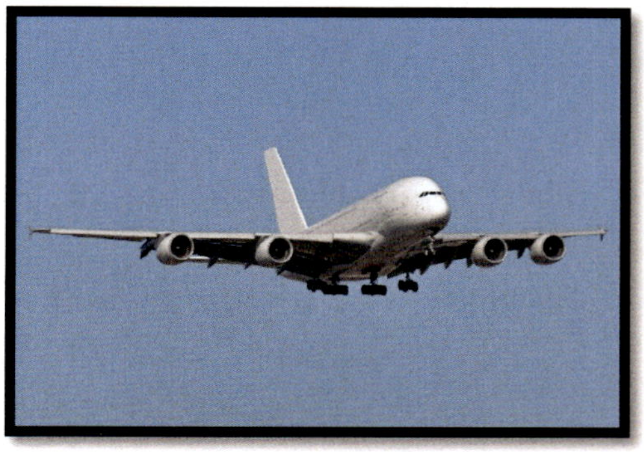

4-3-2. FIRST AID KIT CONTENTS – REQUIRED BY FAA REGULATION

(Example) MedAire's FAK - Meets the Requirements of CFR 121.803(c) (1)

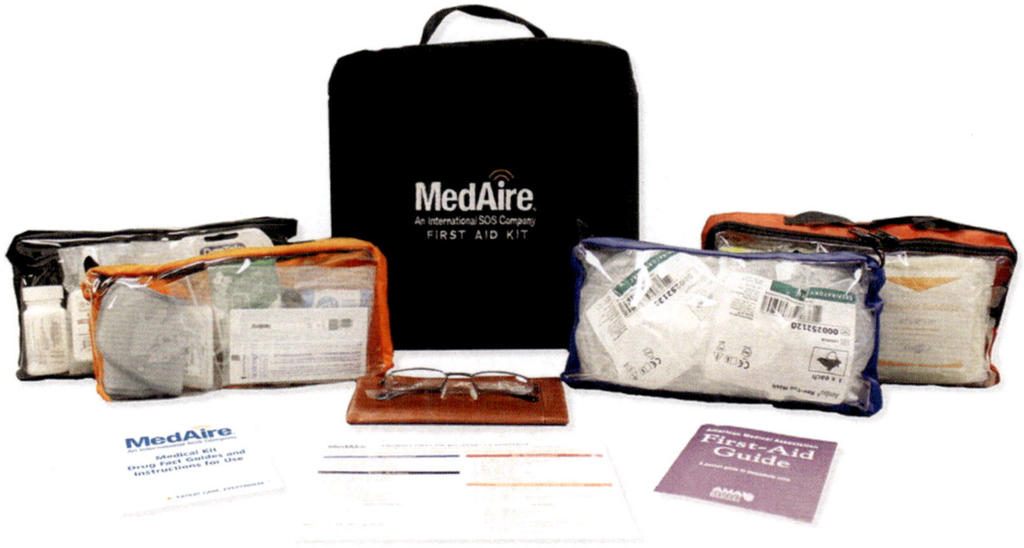

MedAire, First Aid Kit (FAK)

The MedAire FAK includes all the required FAA mandated supplies listed under CFR Title 14, part 121.803 but also contains some extra items for the attending volunteer such as reading glasses (pictured above). Included in the MedAire FAK is a list of its contents for easy reference. FAKs can be customized to the airline's preference, the required supplies are listed below:

MEDAIRE FAK CONTENTS

- ☑ Adhesive bandage compresses, 1-inch (16)
- ☑ Antiseptic swabs (20)
- ☑ Ammonia inhalants (10)
- ☑ Bandage compresses, 4-inch (8)
- ☑ Triangular bandage compresses, 40-inch (5)
- ☑ Arm splint, non-inflatable
- ☑ Leg splint, non-inflatable
- ☑ Roller bandage, 4-inch (4)
- ☑ Adhesive tape, 1-inch standard roll (2)
- ☑ Bandage scissors (U.S. Government Publishing Office, 2015d)

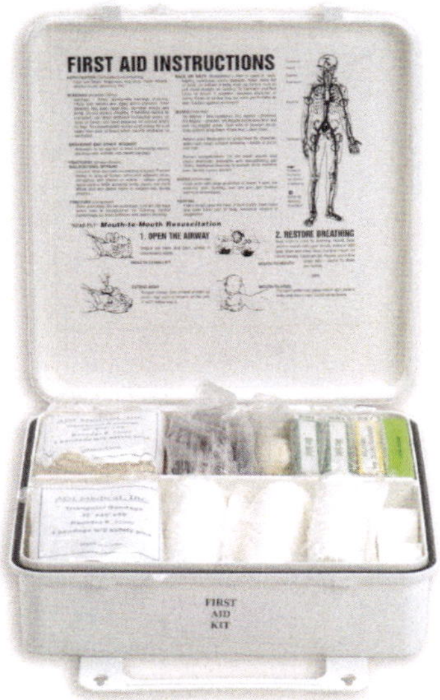

MedAire, First Aid Kit (FAK)

Note:

1. **Depending on the size of aircraft, up to (4) FAKs may be required on each flight.**
2. **The arm and leg splints might be stored outside of the kit's enclosure.**

4-3-3. AIRCRAFT FIRST AID KIT (AFAK) CONTENTS – FOR BUSINESS AND COMMERICAL USE

***(Example)* MedAire's AFAK - Meets the Requirements of CFR 121.803(c) (1)**

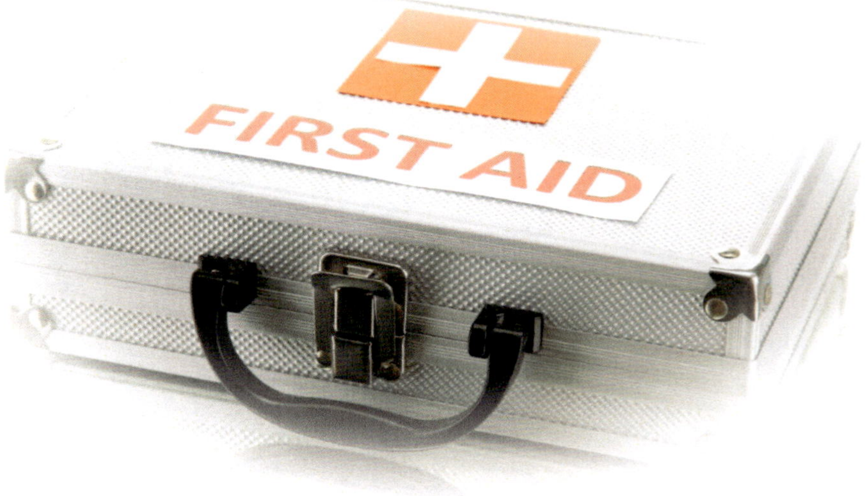

MEDAIRE AFAK CONTENTS

Inside Lid Pocket

Biohazard Bag
Contents Card
Germicidal disinfectant wipe
Ground/air visual code guide
Poly tamper seals
MedLink patch checklist

Inside Perimeter

Dental emergency kit
Ladder splint
Arm board
First Aid record sheet
First Aid handbook
EpiPen (Rx kit)

Blue Airway Pouch

CPR pocket mask with oxygen inlet
Manual suction device
Gloves, non-latex
N95 particle mask
Surgical mask

Red Wound Pouch

Triangular bandages with safety pins
Adhesive strips, 1"
Tape, 1"
Gauze pads, 4" X 4"
Bandage scissors
Gloves, non-latex
Antiseptic towelettes
Gauze bandages, 4" roll
Burn dressings, 4" X 4"
Abdominal gauze pads, 5" X 9"
Adhesive Wound Closures

Orange Assessment Pouch

Emergency Survival Blanket
Stethoscope
Blood pressure cuff
Thermometer, digital
Tweezers

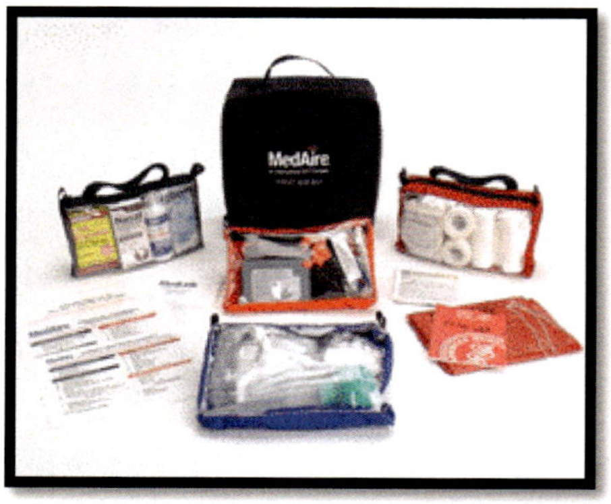

MedAire - Aircraft First Aid Kit (AFAK)

Black Medications Pouch

Cimetidine, 200-mg tabs
Instant cold pack
Glucose 15GM tube (Rx kit)
Nitroglycerin tabs, 0.4 mg (Rx kit)
Oxymetazoline HCL, 0.05% nasal spray
Antacid tablets
Acetaminophen, 500-mg tablets
Ammonia inhalants
Diphenhydramine, 25-mg
Bacitracin ointment
Aspirin, 325-mg tablets
Loperamide HCL, 2-mg tablets
Prednisone, 20-mg tablets (Rx kit)
Water germicidal tablets to treat water
Drinking water packets
Phenazopyridine, 200-mg (Campbell, 2007, pp. 166-167)

4-3-4. FAA REQUIRED EMK OR EEMK CONTENTS

EMK Contents	Quantity
Sphygmomanometer	1
Stethoscope	1
Airways, oropharyngeal (3 sizes): 1 pediatric, 1 small adult, 1 large adult or equivalent	3
Self-inflating manual resuscitation device with 3 masks (1 pediatric, 1 small adult, 1 large adult or equivalent)	1:3
CPR mask (3 sizes), 1 pediatric, 1 small adult, 1 large adult, or equivalent	3
IV Admin Set: Tubing w/ 2 Y connectors	1
Alcohol sponges	2
Adhesive tape, 1-inch standard roll adhesive	1
Tape scissors	1 pair
Tourniquet	1
Saline solution, 500 cc	1
Protective non-permeable gloves or equivalent	1 pair
Needles (2-18 ga., 2-20 ga., 2-22 ga., or sizes necessary to administer required medications)	2 each
Syringes (1-5 cc, 2-10 cc, or sizes necessary to administer required medications)	4
Analgesic, non-narcotic, tablets, 325 mg	4
Antihistamine tablets, 25 mg	4
Antihistamine injectable, 50 mg, (single dose ampule or equivalent)	2
Atropine, 0.5 mg, 5 cc (single dose ampule or equivalent)	2
Aspirin tablets, 325 mg	4
Bronchodilator, inhaled (metered dose inhaler or equivalent)	1
Dextrose, 50%/50 cc injectable, (single dose ampule or equivalent)	1
Epinephrine 1:1000, 1 cc, injectable, (single dose ampule or equivalent)	2
Epinephrine 1:10,000, 2 cc, injectable, (single dose ampule or equivalent)	2
Lidocaine, 5 cc, 20 mg/ml, injectable (single dose ampule or equivalent)	2
Nitroglycerin tablets, 0.4 mg	10
Basic instructions for use of the drugs in the kit	1

Table 5, FAA Required EMK Contents (U.S. Government Publishing Office, 2015d)

An Airbus A380 Only Requires (1) EMK

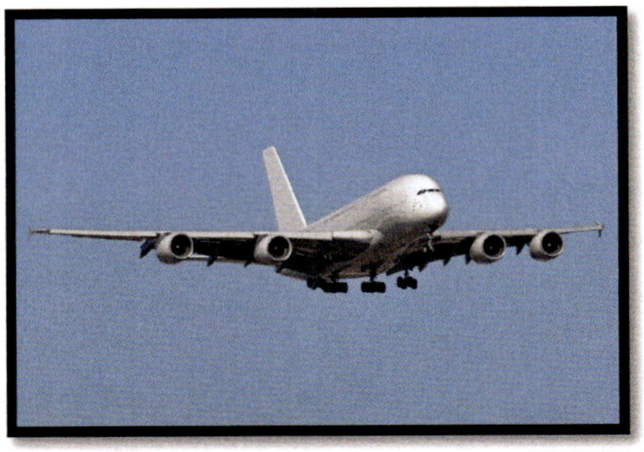

4-3-5. MEDAIRE EMERGENCY MEDICAL KIT (EMK) – COMMERCIAL AIRLINE EXAMPLE

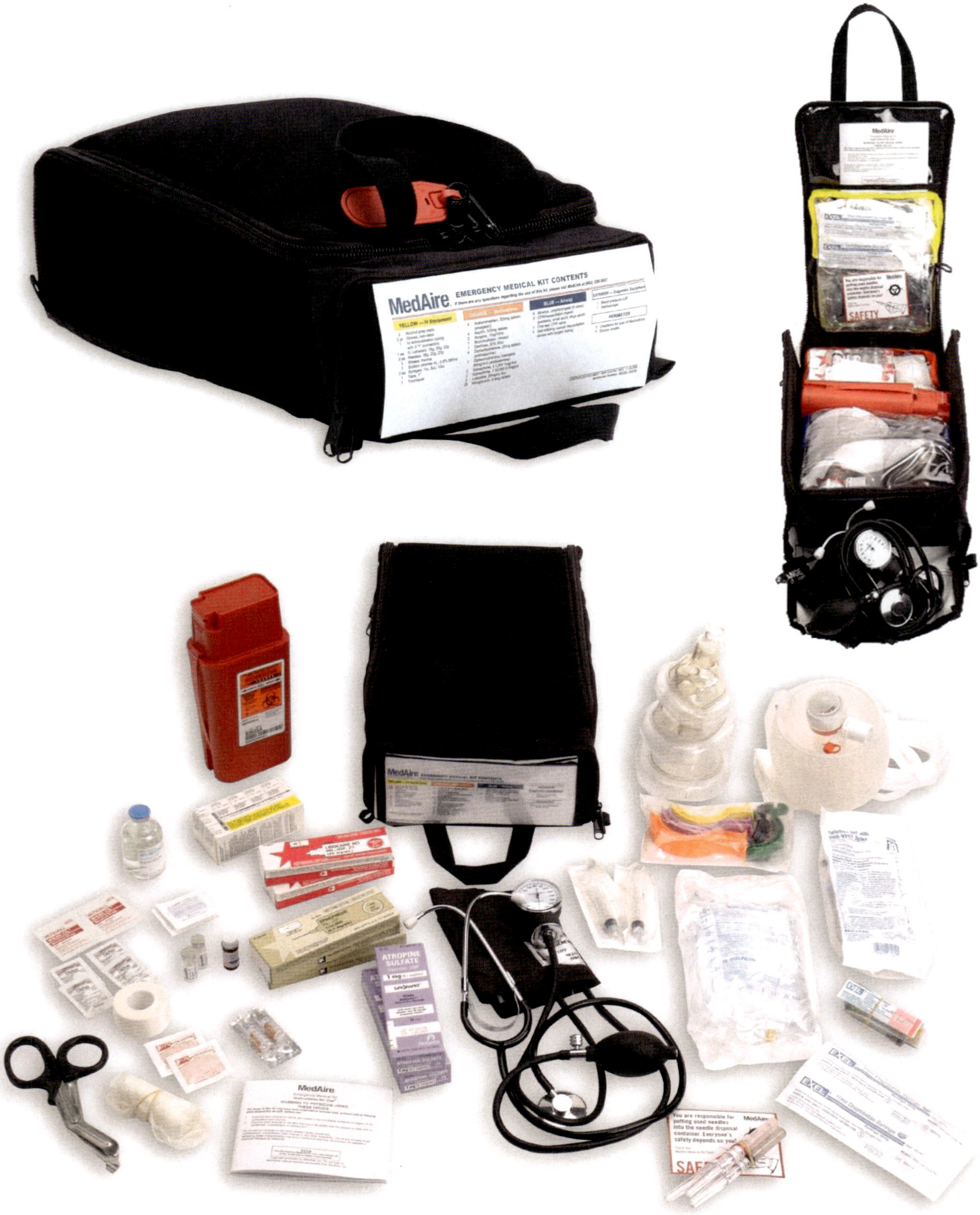

MedAire Commercial Airline Emergency Medical Kit (EMK)

Contents will Vary Due to Product Revisions and Customer Orders - MedAire's EMK Meets the Requirements of CFR 121.803(c) (3)

4-3-6. MEDAIRE EMERGENCY MEDICAL KIT (EMK) CONTENTS

MedAire's EMK - Meets the Requirements of CFR 121.803(c) (3)

(*EXAMPLE*) MEDAIRE EMK CONTENTS FOR BUSINESS AVIATION

1) Right Exterior Pouch
Sharps Container

2) Top Exterior Pouch
Abdominal Pad, sterile
Butterfly bandages
Benzoin tincture
Dressing, sterile 4" X 4"
Gauze, 4" roll
Gloves, non-latex
Knuckle bandages
Pads, non-adherent
Pads, petrolatum gauze
Wound closure strips, 1/4" X 4" (10 pk)
Wound closure strips, 1/2" X 4" (6 pk)

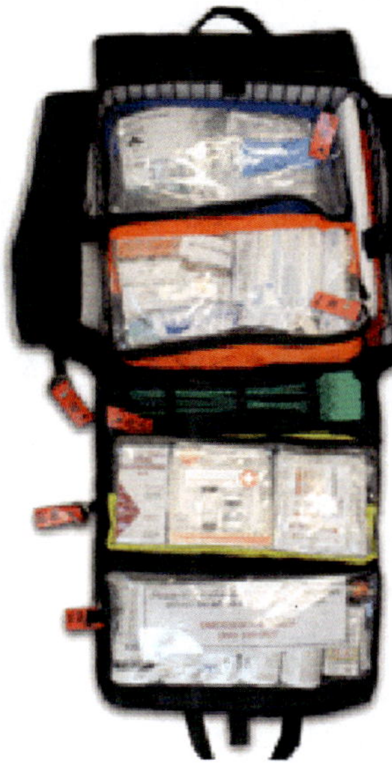

MedAire – Emergency Media Kit (EMK)

3) Left Exterior Pouch
Bloodstopper compression bandages
Gauze rolls, 2.25" and 4.5"
Tape, 1"
Trauma shears

Upper Lid

4) Top Compartment / Black Pouch
Antacid, 420-mg tablets
Ciprofloxacin, 500-mg UD tablets
Diphenhydramine, 50-mg UD tablets
Doxycycline. 100-mg tablets
Fluconazole, 50-mg
Ibuprofen, 200-mg
Metronidazole, 500-mg tablets
Nitroglycerin, 0.4-mg sublingual tablets

5) Middle Compartment / Yellow Pouch
Cephalexin, 500-mg tablets
Ciprofloxacin, ophthalmic solution (eye drops)
Epinephrine auto-injector
First aid thermal blanket
Loperamide HCL, 2-mg tablets
Dimenhydrinate, 50-mg
Oral rehydration salts
Phenylephrine, 10-mg tablets
Sulfamethoxazole / trimethoprim, 800/160-mg tablets

Main Compartment

6) Upper/Blue Pouch
AeroChamber inhaler
IV catheters, 18g (needle safe)
IV catheters, 20g (needle safe)
IV administration tubing with 2 "Y" connectors
IV start kit
N95 mask
Surgical masks

7) Lower/Orange Pouch
Dressings, sterile, 4" X 4"
Gauze, 4" roll
Germicidal tablets for water treatments (25 qt)
Gloves, surgical, sterile
Glucose gel
Instrument tray, all purpose
Needle holder
Povidone-iodine solution
SAM splint
Scalpels, #11
Splash shield
Wound cleanser, 100 mL
Non-latex gloves

Perimeter / Lower Straps
Splint / Trauma dressing

8) Top Zippered Compartment (Includes 9-12)

9) Top Pouch
Ethilon sutures, 3-0 and 5-0
Vicryl suture, 4-0

10) Middle Pouch
20-cc syringe

11) Lower Pouch
18-g, 20-g, and 25-g needles (needle safe)
10-cc and 3-cc syringes
1-cc syringe with 27-g needle (needle safe)
Butterfly infusion sets, 21-g (needle safe)

12) Velcro Sleeve Hidden Pouch
Biohazard bag, germicidal disinfectant wipe
Waterjel burn dressings, 2" X 6"
Directions for use of medications
Content card (Campbell 2007, pp. 168-169)

4-3-7. ENHANCED EMERGENCY MEDICAL KIT (EEMK) – COMMERCIAL AIRLINES

***(Example)* MedAire's EEMK - Meets the Requirements of CFR 121.803(c) (3)**

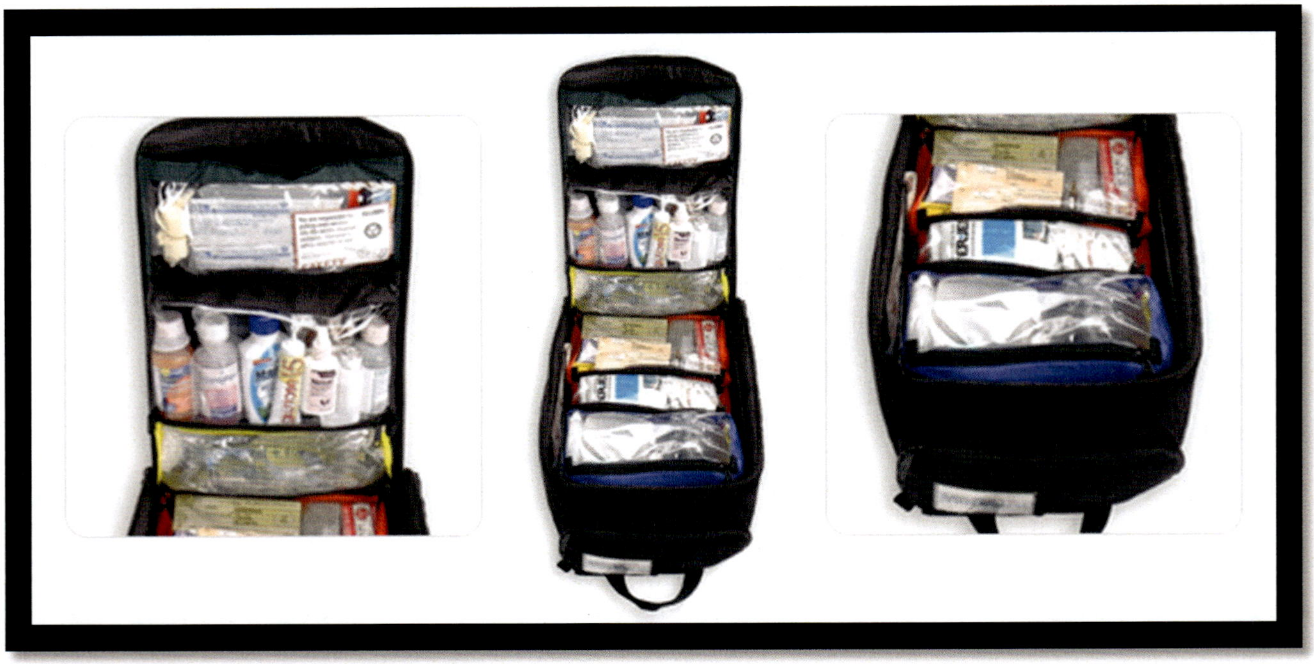

MedAire, Enhanced Emergency Medical Kit (EEMK)

The EMK may also be called the EEMK on airlines that specifically upgrade the components and supplies within the kit. The EEMK is exclusively carried on commercial aircraft and is generally used in conjunction with the EMK or FAK. The EEMK will carry all the contents in the EMK with additional medications and equipment. Many EEMKs are customized to each individual airline's needs, therefore it is difficult to list the contents. The standard procedure for flight crews is to first provide the off-duty EMS professional with the FAK and if that is inadequate in terms of medical equipment and contents, the EEMK will be provided but only if off-duty EMS professionals properly identifies themselves as a medical professional and the flight crew has approved the use of the EEMK. "The EEMK includes medications and other equipment that should be used only by licensed medical professionals, for this reason, flight attendants are not normally trained to use the kit" (Campbell 2007, p. 171).

4-3-8. MEDAIRE ENHANCED EMERGENCY MEDICAL KIT (EEMK) – COMMERCIAL AIRLINES

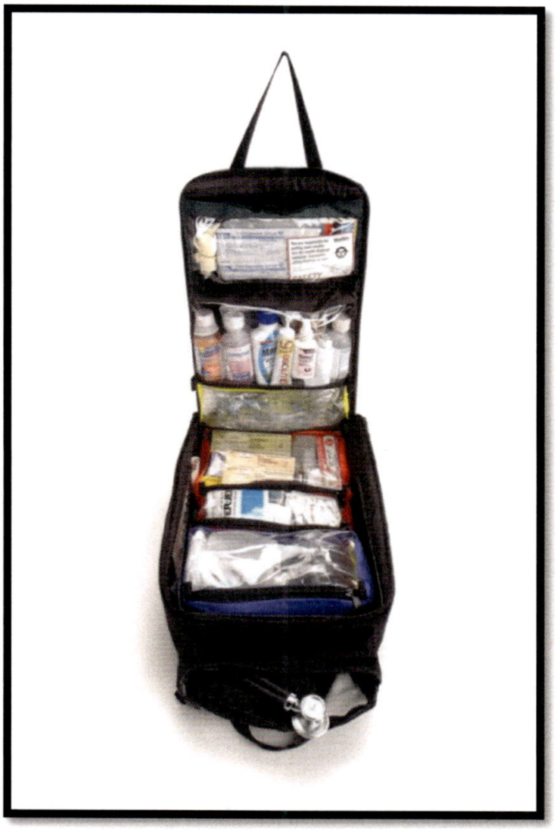

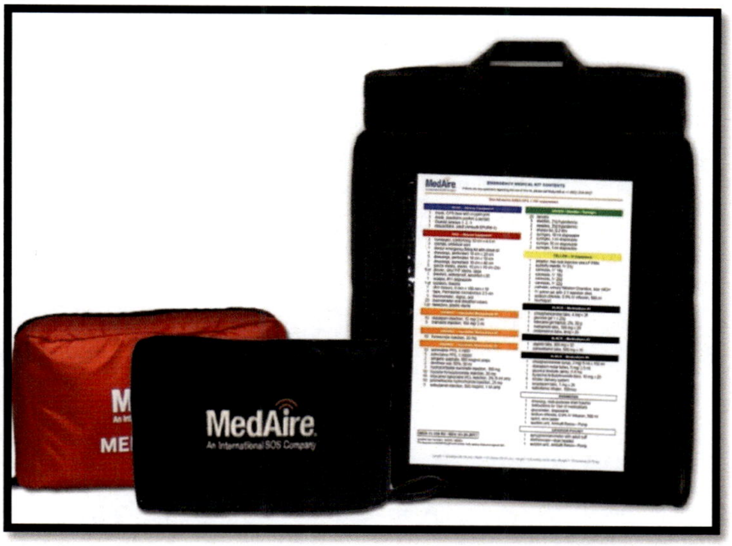

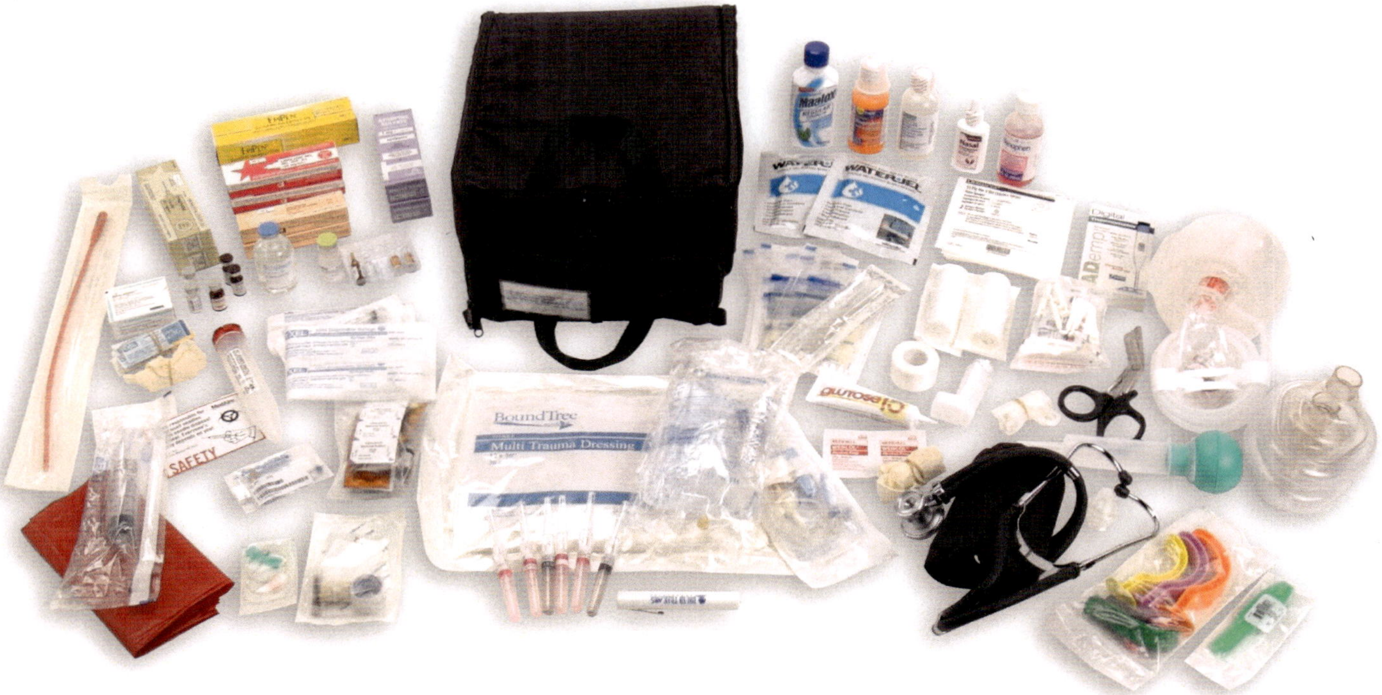

MedAire Commercial Airline Enhanced Emergency Medical Kit (EEMK)

Contents will Vary Due to Product Revisions and Customer Orders - MedAire's EEMK Meets the Requirements of CFR 121.803(c) (3)

4-3-9. SUPPLIERS OF EMK'S AND EEMK'S - MEDAIRE AND BANYAN

There are only a handful of companies that supply in-flight medical kits to commercial airlines. Two of the main suppliers within the United States include MedAire Inc. and Banyan STAT KITS. MedAire serves 115 airlines around the world with a combination of its FAKs, EMKs, and EEMKs and/or the Medlink in-flight medical advisory service. Banyan STAT KITS provides EMKs and EEMKs to its airline partners but does not provide a medical advice service. If you are curious which medical kits will be on your next flight, American, Frontier, Southwest, and United Airlines equip their aircraft with EMKs and EEMKs from Banyan STAT KITS, the remaining airlines use MedAire or another vendor.

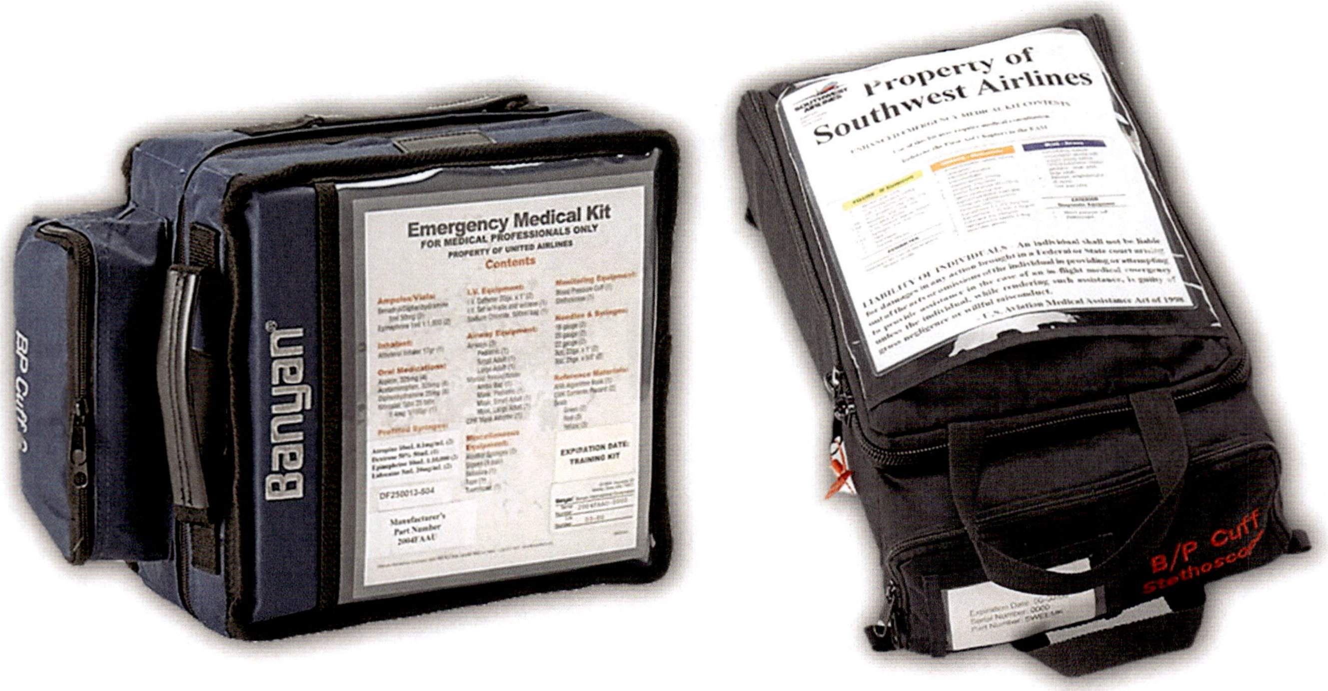

Banyan STAT KITS – United Airlines EEMK and Southwest Airlines EEMK

4-3-10. MEDAIRE UNIVERSAL PRECAUTION KIT (UPK)

According to the International Civil Aviation Organization (ICAO), "one or two universal precaution kits (UPK) should be carried on aircraft that are required to operate with at least one cabin crew member. Additional kit(s) should be made available at times of increased public health risk. Such kits may be used to clean up any potentially infectious body contents such as blood, urine, vomit, and feces and to protect the cabin crew members who are assisting potentially infectious cases of suspected communicable disease" (ICAO, 2017, p. 3). There is currently no regulation that requires UPKs on commercial aircraft. The UPK consists of the following items:

1. Dry powder that can convert small liquid spill into a sterile granulated gel
2. Germicidal disinfectant for surface cleaning
3. Skin wipes
4. Face/eye mask (separate or combined)
5. Gloves (disposable)
6. Protective apron

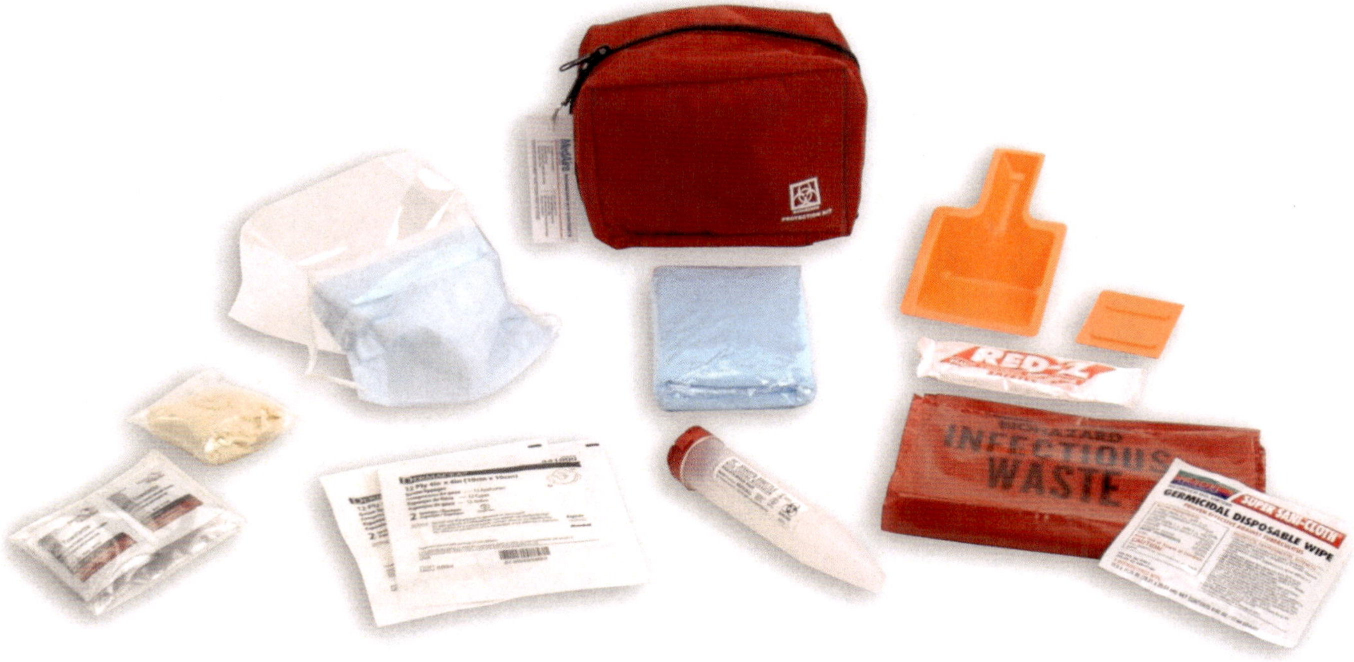

MedAire Universal Precaution Kit (UPK)

4-4. LUFTHANSA DOCTORS KIT – EXCEEDS FAA & EASA REGULATIONS

Doctors Kit

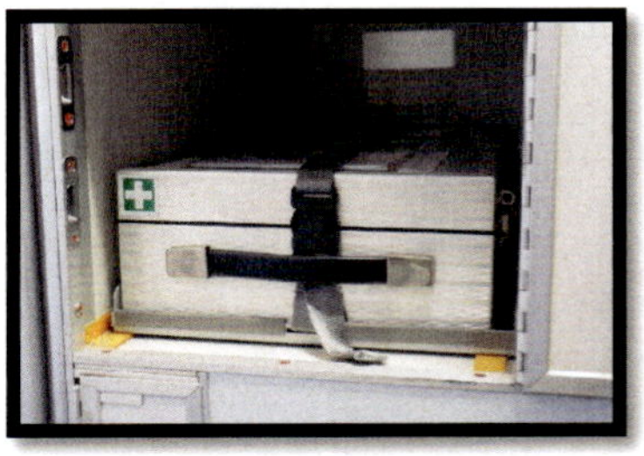

The Lufthansa Doctors Kit will contain more advanced medical equipment such as endotracheal tubes/laryngoscope and additional medications that may not be carried in the EU version of the EMK or FAK depending on each airline. The Doctor's Kit may contain narcotics such as morphine which are regulated to a higher degree than the drugs within the EMK/EEMK (Gabel, et al., 2011).

4-5. MEDAIRE OPTIONAL ADD-ON KITS FOR AIRLINES

→ Universal Precaution Kit (UPK)……………………………………………………

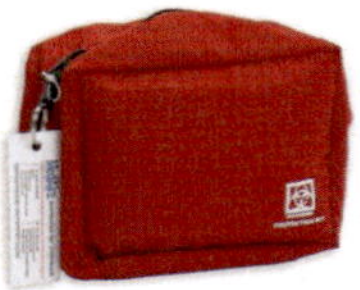

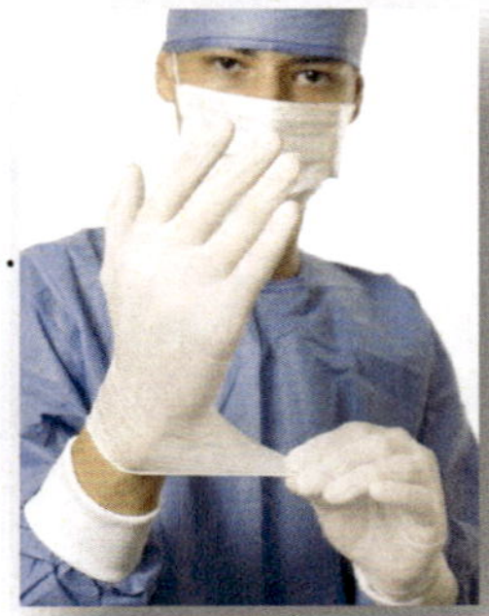

→ Pediatrician Kit……………………………………

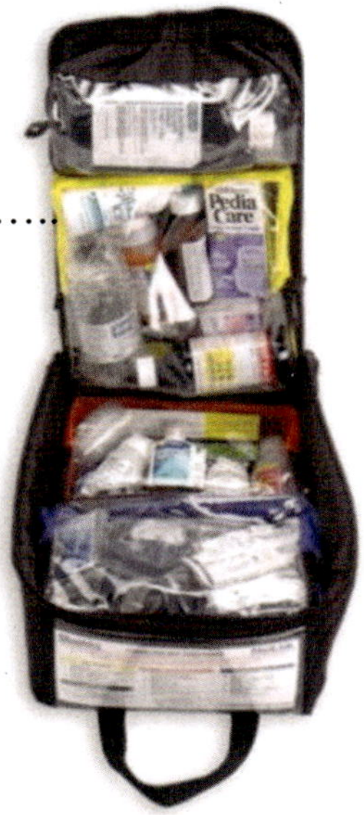

→ Passenger Restraint Kit……

→ EpiPen (epinephrine auto injector)……………………………………………………

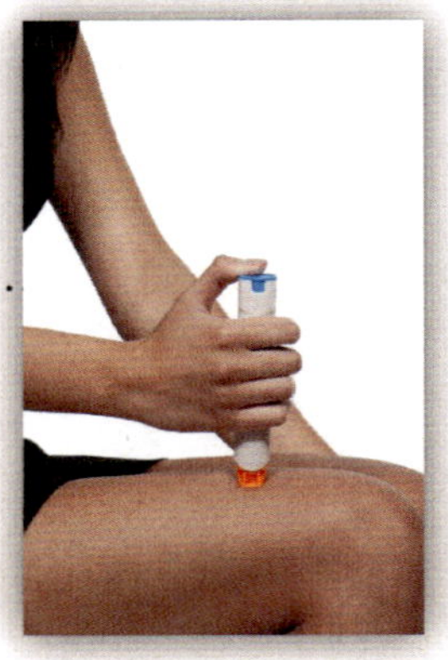

→ Telemedicine Device Screen………..………..…

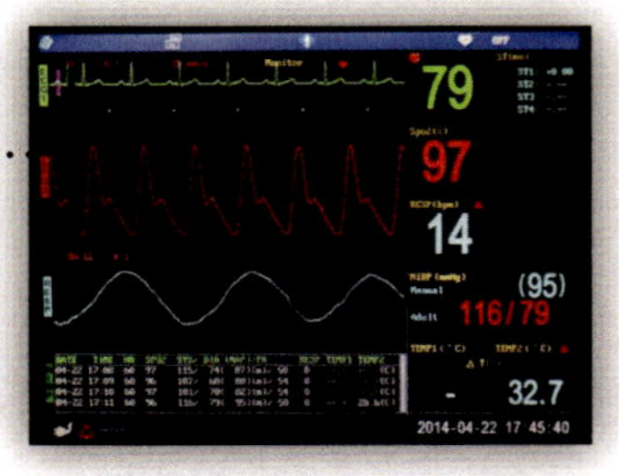

4-6. ACCESS TO EMKS & MEDICAL IDENTIFICATION MAY BE REQUIRED

"Flight Attendants should grant access to the equipment only to trained crewmembers or to other persons qualified and trained in the use of emergency medical equipment. The decision to allow passengers to assist another passenger and have access to medical equipment is up to the air carrier and its agents" (Federal Aviation Administration, 2006, p. 5).

Crewmembers may ask for the off-duty EMS professional's proof of credentials before assistance can be rendered or medical equipment may be obtained. Identification in the form of a professional business card may suffice, or crewmembers may want to see the volunteer's state issued medical credential. During stressful incidents, crewmembers may take the off-duty EMS professionals word in trust if no identification is available; if there is a disagreement between the flight crew and the volunteer, the captain will make the final decision.

4-6-1. WHO IS CONSIDERED MEDICALLY TRAINED BY U.S. STANDARDS?

The term "**medically trained individual**" includes:

> "Any persons who is licensed, certified, or otherwise qualified to provide medical care in a State, including a physician, nurse, physician assistant, paramedic, and emergency medical technician" (House of Representatives, 1998, p. 3).

Crewmembers may ask for the off-duty EMS professional's proof of credentials before assistance can be rendered or medical equipment may be obtained. Identification in the form of a professional business card may suffice, or crewmembers may want to see the volunteer's state issued medical credential. During stressful incidents, crewmembers may take the off-duty EMS professionals word in trust if no identification is available; if there is a disagreement between the flight crew and the volunteer, the captain will make the final decision.

Chapter Notes

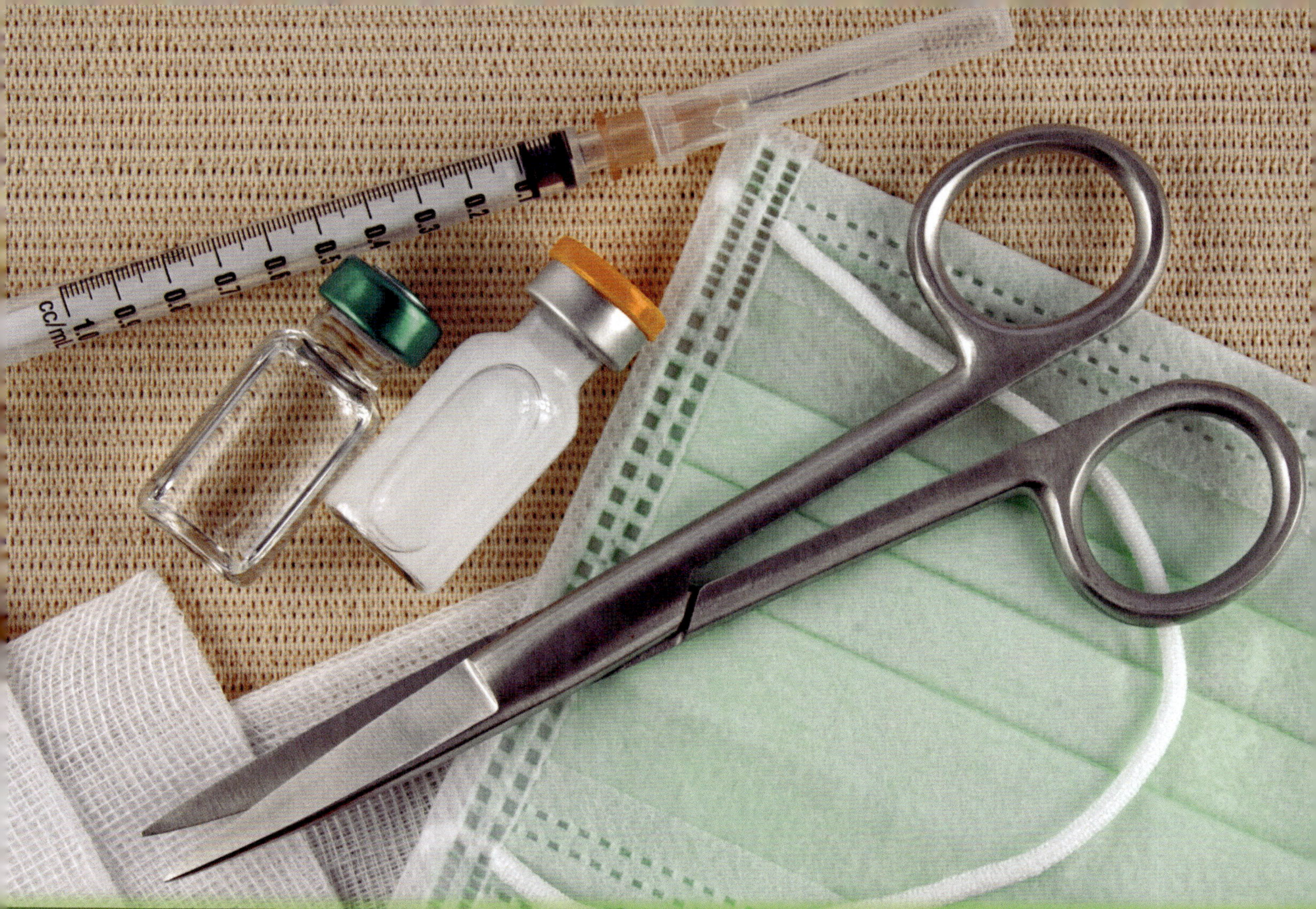

Chapter 5

Medications & Medical Oxygen

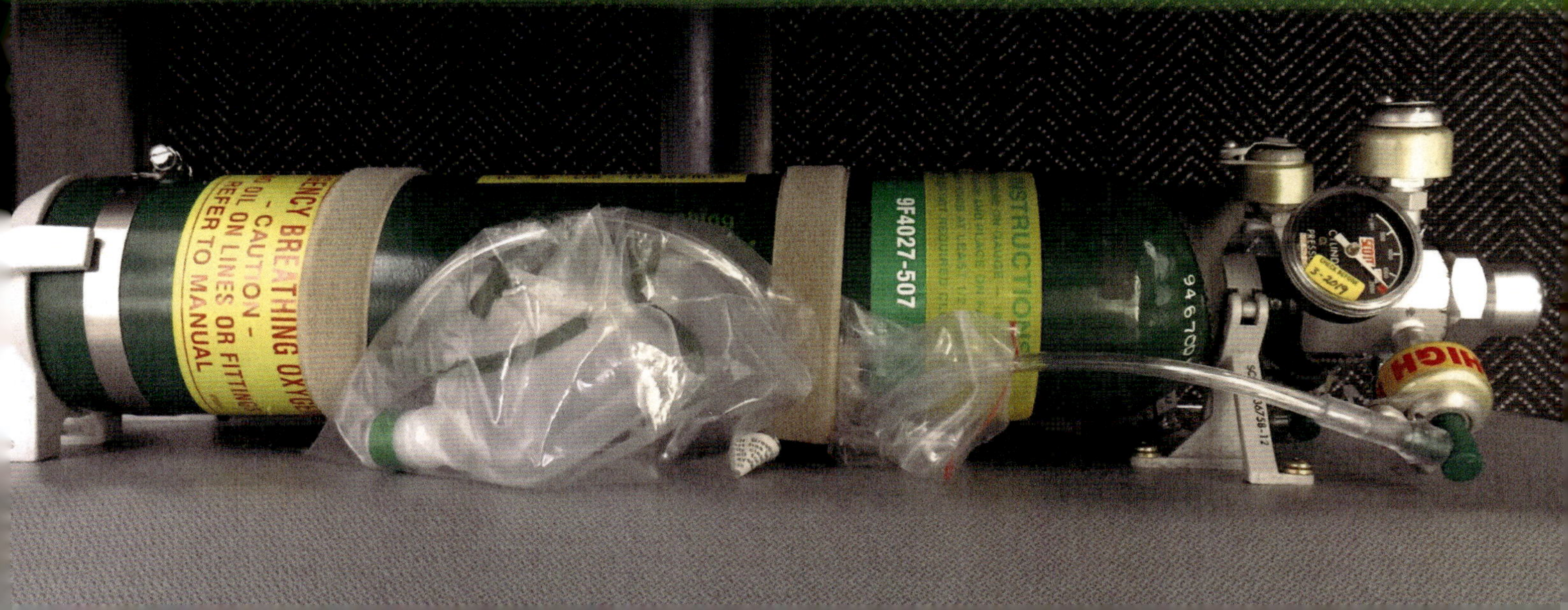

CHAPTER 5: HIGHLIGHTS – MEDICATIONS & MEDICAL OXYGEN

- **Medications Available for IFMEs on Commercial Aircraft**
  - ☑ ESAS Regulations Allow for More Medications than Required
  - ☑ EASA and Other Territories Allow for More Restricted Medications
  - ☑ Comparison of Required EMK Drugs for Different Airlines
  - ☑ Lufthansa Doctors Kit
  - ☑ Top Three Medications used in IFMEs
- **Emergency Oxygen Use In-Flight**
  - ☑ Aviation Oxygen Bottles Primarily used for Rapid Decompression Emergency
  - ☑ Types of Oxygen Tanks and Regulators
  - ☑ Oxygen Delivery Options
  - ☑ Low Flow or High Flow Options
  - ☑ Changing of an Oxygen Regulator is Prohibited In-Flight
- **Dangers of Oxygen Use In-Flight**
  - ☑ Use Within 10 feet of an AED

5-1. MEDICATION AVAILABLE FOR IFME ON COMMERCIAL AIRCRAFT

If airlines would like to carry more medical equipment than required by FAA and EASA regulations, they are free to do so. Medications that are restricted in the U.S. (i.e., narcotics - morphine) must be ordered directly through a vendor who currently has a valid Drug Enforcement Administration (DEA) registration certificate on file (Federal Aviation Administration, 2006). Many airlines around the world order customized EEMKs from MedAire with additional medications and supplies not required by the FAA and EASA; additional components such as the EpiPen epinephrine auto-injector can be added to the kits (Alves, 2015). The FAA requires EMKs (or EEMKs) to contain at a minimum the following medications:

Standard EMK Medication Components - Includes I.V. Equipment and Syringes/Needles

- ☑ Analgesic, non-narcotic, tablets, 325 mg
- ☑ Antihistamine tablets, 25 mg
- ☑ Antihistamine injectable, 50 mg, single dose ampule
- ☑ Atropine, 0.5 mg, 5 cc, single dose ampule
- ☑ Aspirin tablets, 325 mg
- ☑ Bronchodilator, inhaled, metered dose inhaler
- ☑ Dextrose, 50%/50 cc injectable, single dose ampule
- ☑ Epinephrine 1:1000, 1 cc, injectable, single dose ampule
- ☑ Epinephrine 1:10,000, 2 cc, injectable, single dose ampule
- ☑ Lidocaine, 5 cc, 20 mg/ml, injectable, single dose ampule
- ☑ Nitroglycerine tablets, 0.4 mg
- ☑ Basic instructions for use of the drugs in the EMK/EEMK" (FAA, 2006, p 2)

5-1-1. EASA AND OTHER COUNTRIES REQUIRE MORE MEDICATIONS IN EMK'S AND DOCTORS KITS

The FAA and EASA require specific minimum requirements for their EMK or equivalent kits. Any airline may carry a larger selection of medications within its EMKs and this is generally seen primarily with long-haul aircraft where flights involve crossing vast oceans. Lufthansa provides a more sophisticated Doctor's Kit for their long-haul flights which includes several more medications than the standard EMK or EEMK.

Note: Some international airline carriers are removing Diazepam from their EEMKs and Doctors Kits because of difficulties in supplying this controlled substance.

Continue to Next Page

5-2. REQUIRED EMK DRUGS FOR DIFFERENT AIRLINES

Comparison of Required EMK Drugs for Different Enforcement Authorities and Airlines

FAA	European EASA	Air Canada	Japan Airlines	Qantas Airways
Antihistamine tablet	Adrenocorticosteroid	Aspirin	Aspirin	Adrenaline
Antihistamine injectable	Antiemetic (metoclopramide)	Lorazepam	Atropine	Anginine
Aspirin tablet	Antihistamine	Atropine	Aminophylline injectable	Aspirin
Atropine ampule	Antispasmodic (hyoscine)	Diphenhydramine hydrochloride	Berberine	Atropine
Dextrose injectable	Aspirin	Bicarbonate	Chlorpheniramine tablets	Benztropine
Epinephrine injectable	Atropine	Dextrose	Chinese herb medicine	Benzylpenicillin
External automated defibrillator	Bronchodilator	Epinephrine	Epinephrine	Diazepam
Inhaled bronchodilator	Digoxin	Glucagon	Diazepam injectable	Furosemide
Lidocaine	Diuretic (furosemide)	Gravol	Dopamine injectable	Haloperidol
Nitroglycerin tablets	Epinephrine	Haloperidol	Furosemide injectable	Hyoscine
Nonnarcotic analgesic	Hypertonic glucose	Propranolol hydrochloride	Fradiomycin sulfate gauze	Lignocaine
	Major analgesic (nalbuphine)	Instaglucose	Glycerin enema	Loperidol
	Nitroglycerin	Furosemide	Hydrocortisone injectable	Morphine
	Sedative/anticonvulsant (diazepam)	Lidocaine	Isosorbide dinitrate	Naloxone
	Uterine-contracting agent (ergometrine/oxytocin)	Morphine	Lidocaine injectable	Paracetamol suppository
		Nitroglycerin	Methylergometrine injectable	Phenytoin
		Procainamide	Nitroglycerin tablets	Prednisolone
		Solumedrol	Nifedipine capsules	Prochlorperazine
		Tylenol	Pabron Gold	Promethazine
		Diazepam	Ritodrine tablets	Oxytocin
		Albuterol	Scopolamine injectable	Diazepam
			Sodium bicarbonate injectable	Albuterol inhaler
			Sulpyrine injectable	Verapamil
			Terbutaline injectable	

Table 6, Comparison of Required EMK Drugs for Different Enforcement Authorities and Airlines, Source: Sirven, 2006

5-2-1. LUFTHANSA DOCTORS KIT – MEDICATIONS LIST

Some international airlines may carry a Doctor's Kit in addition to the EEMK. The Doctors Kit may have additional medical supplies and/or medications; these kits are generally reserved specifically for physicians for the treatment of life-threatening conditions (Gabel et al., 2011). The Doctor's Kits will contain more advanced medical equipment such as endotracheal tubes/laryngoscope and additional medications that may not be carried in the EMK or the EEMK. The FAA does not require EMKs to carry controlled substances and if airlines choose to carry such items (e.g., diazepam, morphine) they must purchase them through an EMK vender such as MedAire where the vender has a current DEA Registration Certificate on file (AC 121-33b). Additional supplies/medications in the Doctor's Kit may include:

Equipment

- ☑ ETT sizes 3,4,5,6,7.5
- ☑ Laryngoscope with blade size 2.3
- ☑ Hand Held Portable Suction Unit
- ☑ Finger pulse oximeter
- ☑ Blood Sugar test

Medications

- ☑ Akineton ampoule 5 mg/1 ml
- ☑ Aqua pro injection ampoule 150 mg/3 ml
- ☑ Aspirin IV ampoule
- ☑ Bayotensin akut vial
- ☑ Beloc IV ampoule
- ☑ Bronchoparat ampoule
- ☑ Bronchospasmin ampoule .09 mg/1 ml

- ☑ Buscopan ampoule 20 mg/1 ml & suppository
- ☑ Diazepam ampoule 10 mg/2 ml & rectal tube 10 mg
- ☑ Dormicum ampoule 15 mg.3 ml
- ☑ Glucose 40% ampoule 10 ml
- ☑ Ebrantil 50 ampoule/10 ml
- ☑ Haldol-Janssen ampoule 5 mg/1 ml
- ☑ Heparin-Natrium 5000 ratiopharm
- ☑ Isotonic NaCI solution 0.9% 10 ml
- ☑ Jonosteril Freeflex Electrolyte Solution 500 ml (2 units)
- ☑ Ketanest S ampoule 50 mg/2 ml
- ☑ Lasix ampoule 40 mg
- ☑ MCP ratio ampoule 10mg/2 ml
- ☑ Novaminsulfon ratio ampoule 2.5g/5 ml
- ☑ Paracetamol 250 suppository
- ☑ Proagent eye drops
- ☑ Ranitidin ratio pro injection
- ☑ Rectodelt suppository 100 mg
- ☑ Solu-Decortin H ampoule 250 mg
- ☑ Tavegil ampoule 2 mg/5ml
- ☑ Tramal ampoule 100 mg/2 ml
- ☑ Vomacur 150 suppository

5-2-2. MOST COMMON MEDICATIONS USED IN-FLIGHT

Interestingly, the majority of the medications on-board commercial flights are rarely used. The following list includes the top three medications used in-flight (O_2 generally needs an Rx):

1) Oxygen use ....49.9% of cases
2) Intravenous 0.9% saline solution use...... ....5.2% of cases
3) Aspirin use...5.0% of cases (Peterson et al., 2013)

5-3. FLIGHT CREW – AVIATION PORTABLE OXYGEN BOTTLES

- Oxygen bottles are primarily used for a rapid decompression emergency
- All seated passengers have a 10-minute oxygen supply during rapid decompression
- Portable oxygen bottles are used for first aid treatment of rapid decompression
- Each flight attendant has 15-75 minutes of oxygen at 2-4 LPM
- Oxygen bottles are not intended for routine medical purposes
- Oxygen bottles may be used for IFMEs when no other emergency exists (Gabel et al., 2011)
- Oxygen bottle use - priority given to flight attendants

Airlines must supply the pilots and the cabin crew with emergency oxygen in the event of a rapid decompression emergency in the cabin. Portable oxygen bottles stowed by flight attendants at their stations are intended to provide no less than 15 minutes of oxygen to each flight attendant so they may move about the cabin to assist passengers during a decompression emergency (U. S. Government Publishing Office 2015a). In the event of a rapid decompression, the aircraft must have enough portable oxygen systems available to provide 2% of the passengers with oxygen for the duration of the flight with no less than two portable oxygen systems on every flight. There is no requirement for airlines to specifically carry medical oxygen for the specific purpose of IFMEs. Many airlines will allow the use of the aviation portable oxygen bottles for IFMEs when no other emergency exists.

For IFMEs, passengers are generally given an aviation oxygen bottle with either a nasal cannula or an oxygen mask designed for aviation use. Here are some details about the oxygen bottles:

- ☑ Oxygen fittings may not work with nasal cannula/mask tubing
- ☑ Bag Valve Mask (BVM) / CPR mask tubing may not connect
- ☑ May have to use mask already attached to oxygen bottle
- ☑ High pressure bottle full at 1800 pounds per square inch (PSI)
- ☑ Oxygen regulator is limited to 4 liters per minute (LPM) on most aircraft
- ☑ No high flow (5 LPM or higher) option
- ☑ **DANGER** - Oxygen regulator cannot be removed from bottle in-flight
- ☑ Tank considered empty at 500 PSI

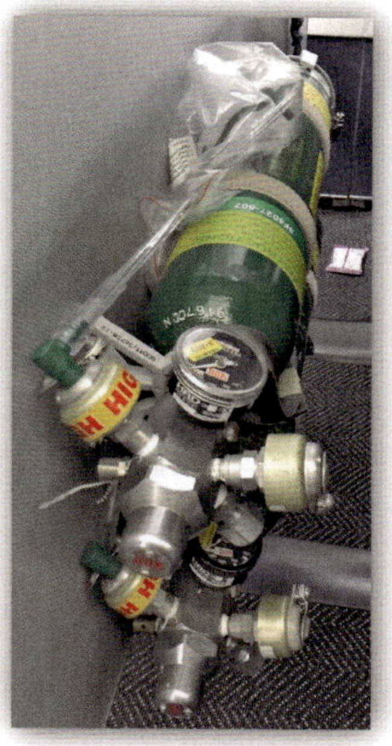

Aviation Portable Oxygen

5-3-1. OXYGEN DELIVERY BY NASAL CANNULA, BVM, OR FACE MASK

Nasal Cannula | **BVM** | **Face Mask**

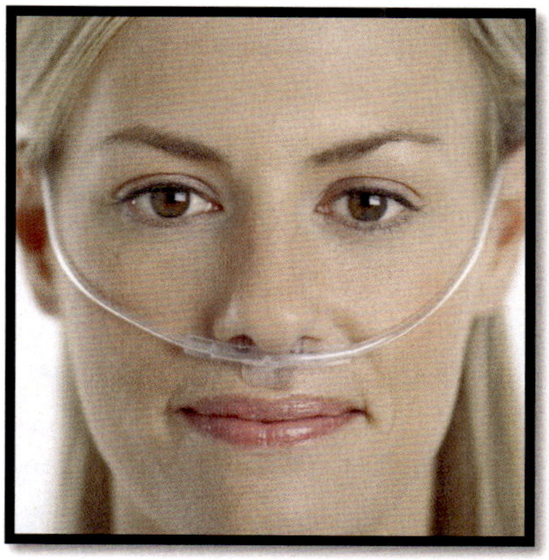

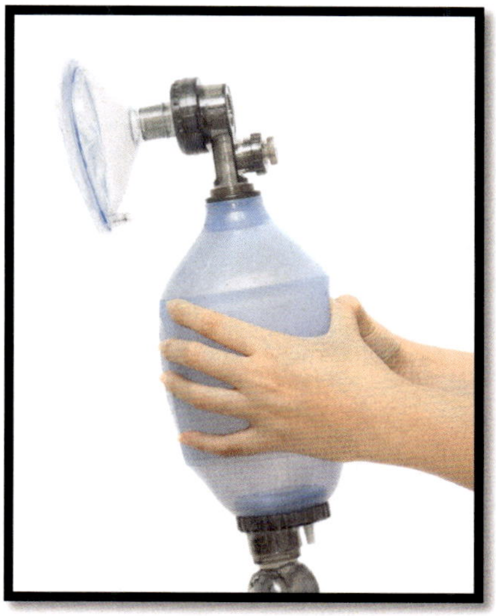

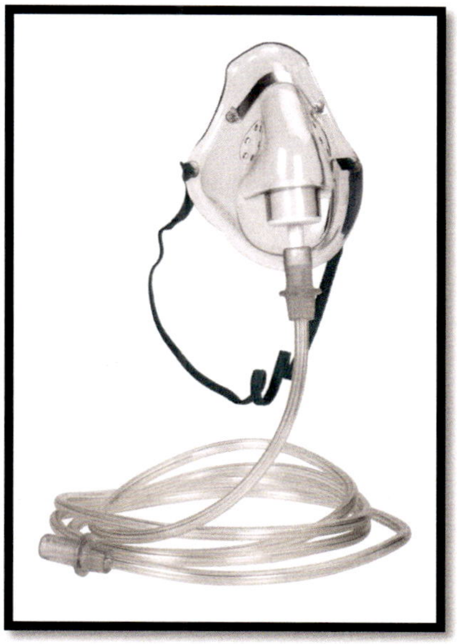

The items pictured above are generally carried on-board commercial aircraft, ask a flight attendant for assistance when requesting oxygen and the related delivery systems.

5-3-2. OXYGEN BOTTLE REGULATOR LIMITS O_2 RATE IN-FLIGHT

EMS professionals are generally accustomed to oxygen systems that have a low flow rate from 1-6 LPM for nasal cannulas and a high flow rate of 7-25 LPM for face masks, BVMs, ETTs, and King tubes. Because the portable oxygen systems on-board aircraft are designed primarily for the flight attendants, the LPM rate is restricted to ensure the oxygen flow will last for the duration of the in-flight emergency. These portable oxygen systems can be used for IFMEs when no other emergency exists. These in-flight portable oxygen systems will generally have 2 flow rates:

- Low flow – 2 LPM
- Med flow – 4 LPM

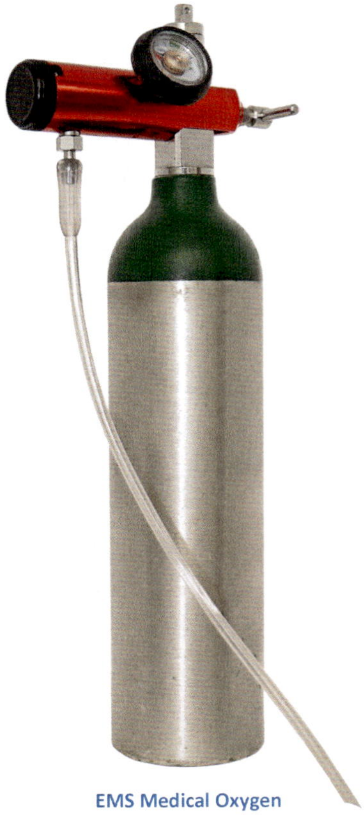

EMS Medical Oxygen

5-3-3. CHANGING OF AN OXYGEN REGULATOR IS PROHIBITED IN-FLIGHT

FAA regulations prohibit the removal of an oxygen regulator from a bottle while in-flight – those providing emergency care must ask a flight attendant for assistance if the O_2 bottle needs to be replaced with a full tank (Federal Aviation Administration, 2006). Aviation O_2 bottles are considered full at 1800 PSI and empty at 500 PSI. If during an IFME an O_2 bottle reaches 500 PSI, continue to use until replaced with a full tank. If no other bottles are available, the regulator shall be changed to the lowest LPM setting to extend the time of remaining O_2. It is advised not to allow the O_2 bottle to completely empty.

5-4. DANGERS OF OXYGEN USE IN-FLIGHT

Note: Oxygen can be explosive in a pressurized environment such as in an aircraft cabin.

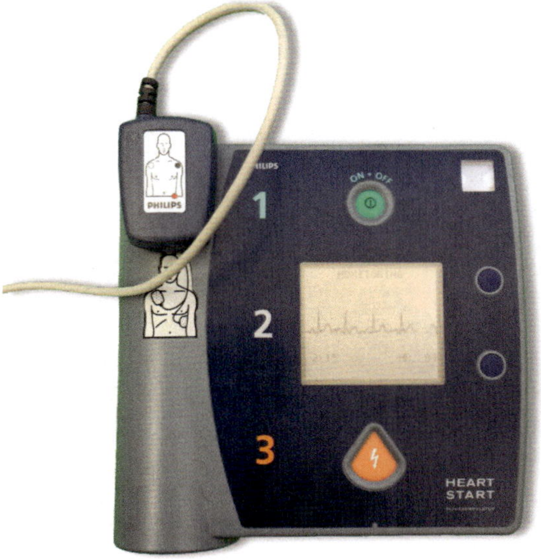

Do not use supplemental oxygen within 10 feet of a patient in cardiac arrest when the AED is being used to deliver a shock (Federal Aviation Administration, 2006). A high concentration of oxygen near a spark in a pressurized environment can be dangerous. The use of an AED as a monitor using a specialized three-lead connection may disable the shock feature and therefore, can be used in the presence of a supplemental oxygen source. (Photo shown with Phillips FR2+ with monitor only attachment).

5-4-1. DANGERS OF LOW FLOW (LESS THAN 6 LPM) O_2 REGULATORS

EMS professionals use medical O_2 on a regular basis when responding to medical calls on the ground. These ground-based O_2 regulators have a low flow rate from 1-6 LPM for nasal cannulas and a high flow rate of 7-25 LPM for face masks, BVMs, ETTs, and King tubes.

During an IFME, the medical use of an aviation O_2 bottle and mask at 2-4 LPM can create a dangerous situation for a patient in distress. The patient may experience a situation where not enough O_2 is being inhaled from the face mask while simultaneously too much carbon dioxide (CO_2) is being re-inhaled from the same mask. With this type of O_2 mask set up, the patient may re-inhale their expired CO_2 making their breathing more labored and their medical condition worse. Ensure that the aviation medical O_2 face mask has proper exhalation ports and is not a non-rebreather mask. In most situations on a conscious patient, it would be best to only use the nasal cannula when delivering an O_2 rate of 2-4 LPM.

Note: Ask the flight attendant for a medical O_2 bottle. Airlines may carry medical grade O_2 bottles and related regulators which will have up to a 25 LPM flow rate.

Chapter Notes

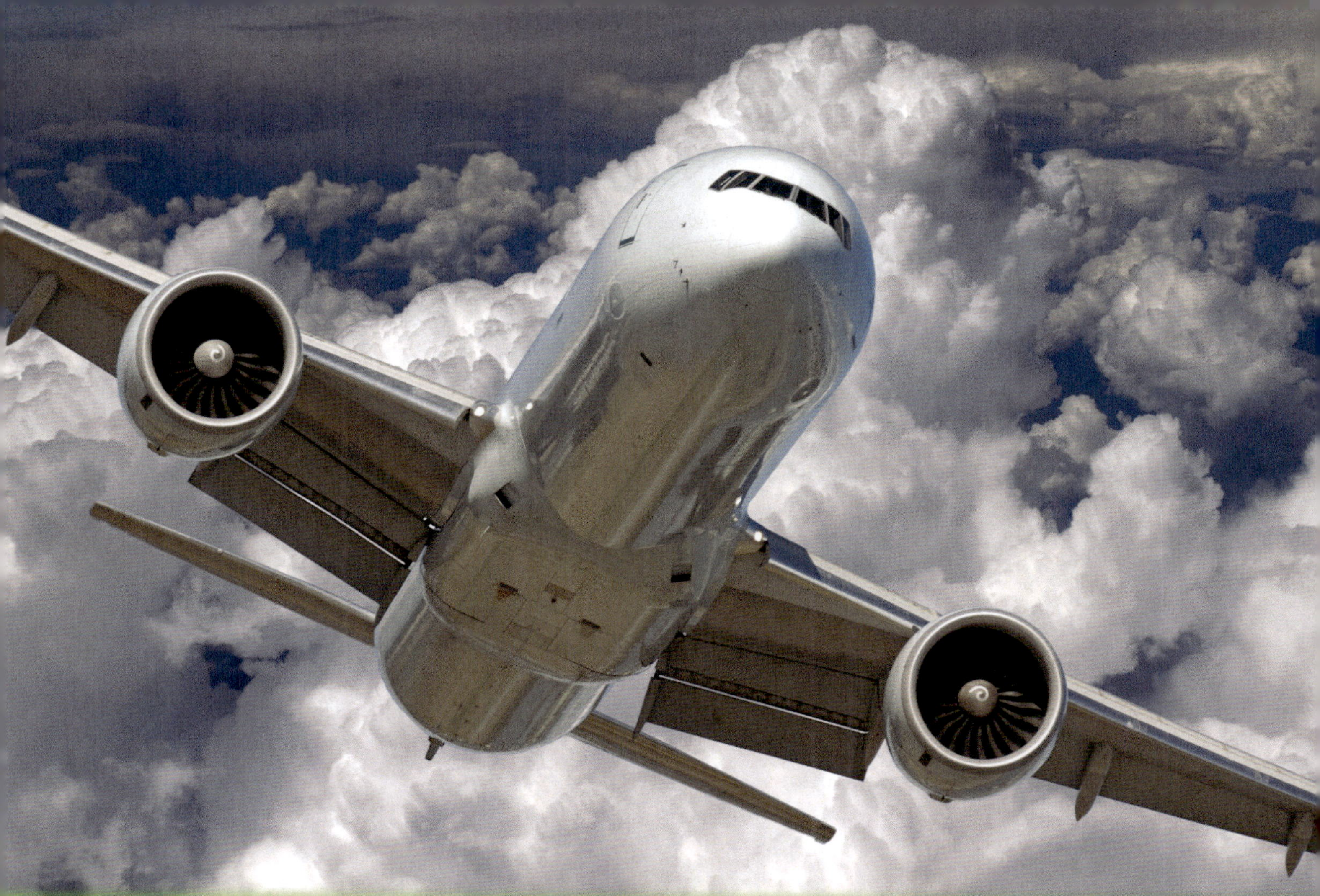

Chapter 6

Aircraft Pressurization Issues

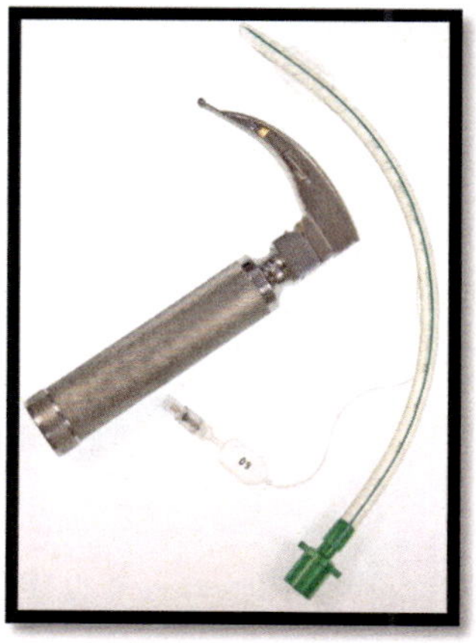

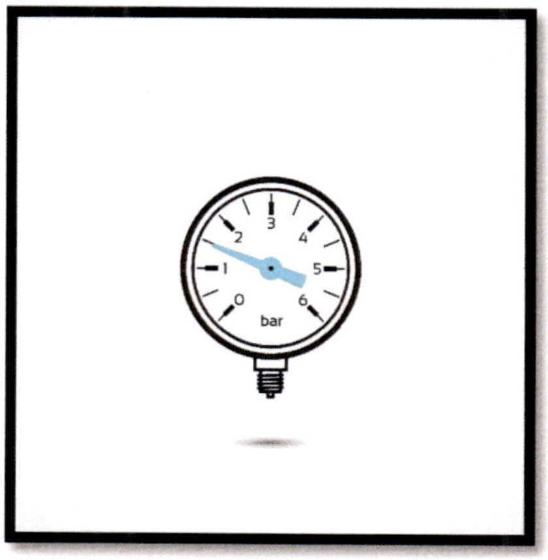

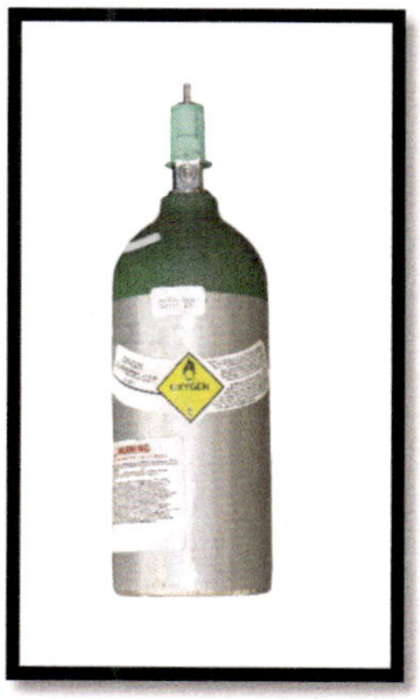

CHAPTER 6: HIGHLIGHTS – AIRCRAFT PRESSURIZATION ISSUES

- **Introduction to the Atmosphere and Aircraft Cabin Pressure**
  - ☑ Dalton's Law Pertaining to Air Travel
  - ☑ Boyle's Law Pertaining to Air Travel
  - ☑ Cabin Pressure vs. Outside Pressure
- **Medical Complications Related to Being In-Flight**
  - ☑ Effects of Flying on the Body
    - Pulse Oximeter
  - ☑ Dehydration
    - Alcohol Consumption
- **Endotracheal Tube Complications at Altitude**
  - ☑ Unable to Maintain Cuff Pressures During Ascents and Descents
  - ☑ Dangerous to Patient if not Constantly Monitored

6-1. INTRODUCTION TO THE ATMOSPHERE AND AIRCRAFT PRESSURIZATION ISSUES

Commercial airlines fly in the portion of earth's atmosphere known as the troposphere, generally between 24,000 feet and 40,000 feet. The troposphere begins at sea level and rises to approximately 50,000 feet where the atmospheric temperature is measured as minus Fahrenheit (F) or Celsius (C) degrees and oxygen levels are insufficient to support life (Campbell, 2007). The atmospheric pressure is greatest at sea level and diminishes as altitude is gained, causing the air to thin. The earth's atmospheric gases as displayed in Figure 7 are primarily comprised of nitrogen (79.08%), oxygen (20.95%), argon (0.93%), carbon dioxide (0.03%), hydrogen (0.00006%), neon (0.0018%), and helium (0.0005%) (Campbell, 2007). All the earth's gasses are considered partial pressures when referred to individually.

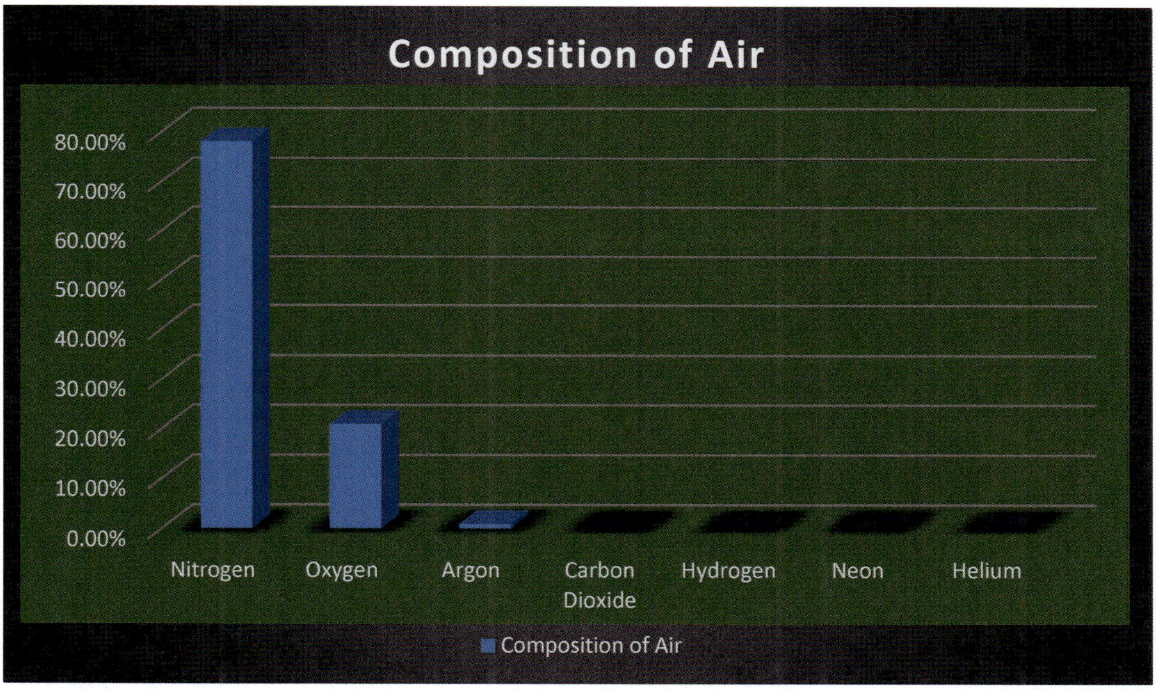

Figure 7, Composition of Air Gases

As altitude increases, atmospheric barometric pressure decreases. As the partial pressure of O_2 decreases with altitude, the percentage of O_2 decreases as well.

At sea level the atmosphere's barometric pressure, which is measured as millimeters of mercury (mmHg), is 760. At 18,000 feet, the pressure is reduced to 380 mmHg, and at 33,700 feet, the pressure is reduced to

190 mmHg (Campbell, 2007). The reduction of atmospheric pressure results in significantly less O_2 levels at altitude which makes an aircraft fuselage a life-support system when above 12,000 feet.

6-1-1. DALTON'S LAW PERTAINING TO AIR TRAVEL

Dalton's law states that the total pressure of a system (a pressurized aircraft cabin) is equal to the sum of the partial pressures within that system (all gases within the aircraft cabin). At sea level the total atmospheric barometric pressure totals 760 mmHg and the partial pressure (20.95%) of O_2 measures 160 mmHg (Chandra & Conry, 2013). When in-flight, a pressurized aircraft (7,874 feet equivalent) at cruising altitude (33,000 feet) would have a reduced O_2 partial pressure of 118 mmHg, or approximately 25% less O_2 by pressure when compared to sea level. For this reason, breathing at altitude becomes more difficult because there is simply less O_2 within the aircrafts cabin. As a comparison, the altitude of Aspen, Colorado, is approximately 7,800 feet above sea level and the average healthy person can ascend to 7,800 feet without difficulty (Chandra & Conry, 2013).

Note: If a patient during an IFME states he/she cannot travel in mountainous regions due to his/her health, the most likely culprit of their in-flight illness may be the lack of O_2 within the cabin.

6-1-2. BOYLE'S LAW PERTAINING TO AIR TRAVEL

Boyle's law states "the volume that a gas occupies is inversely proportional to the surrounding pressure" (Silverman & Gendreau, 2008, p. 2068). In other words, if a container such as a tire was reduced in size by half its volume, the pressure from the air inside the tire would double. For this reason, large off-road tires may only need 25 pounds per square inch (PSI) of air pressure, while narrow tires of the same circumference may need 50 PSI of air pressure to be properly inflated.

Boyles' law is important to air travel because low cabin pressures associated with cruising altitudes can cause the expansion of body gases by 30% (Silverman & Gendreau, 2008). Airline passengers who have had to clear their ears or had abdominal cramps while flying have experienced Boyle's law. Passengers who are scuba divers shall wait at least 24 hours after their last dive before they can safely fly, otherwise they increase their risk for decompression sickness (Silverman & Gendreau, 2008).

The understanding of Boyle's law is critical when using medical equipment that contain air bladders (ETT, BP cuff, air splints, and catheters). The improper use of medical equipment that contain air bladders while in-flight may cause additional unintended injuries to the patient. Overexpansion or under expansion of IFME devices utilized on patients while ascending or descending in an aircraft, has the potential to cause significant injuries. As a general IFME safety precaution, do not use medical equipment that contain air bladders while ascending or descending.

6-1-3. CABIN PRESSURE VS. ATMOSPHERIC PRESSURE

To make air travel safe and comfortable for passengers and crewmembers, aircraft manufacture's design commercial airliners to be pressurized at a consistent altitude just below 8,000 feet. In accordance with FAA regulations, commercial aircraft flying at a cruising altitude will generally maintain cabin pressures at or below 7,874 feet (Chandra & Conry, 2013). New generation aircraft, such as the Boeing 787 Dreamliner, can maintain cabin pressures of 6,000 feet or less at altitude, improving passenger comfort while providing a higher partial percentage of O_2 within the cabin (Rushkin et al., 2008). In addition to pressurizing the cabin, the air is heated and filtered for passenger comfort. The humidity of a pressurized aircraft cabin is very low, often at around 10%, the Boeing 787 Dreamliner has an increased percentage of air humidity within its cabin of around 30%.

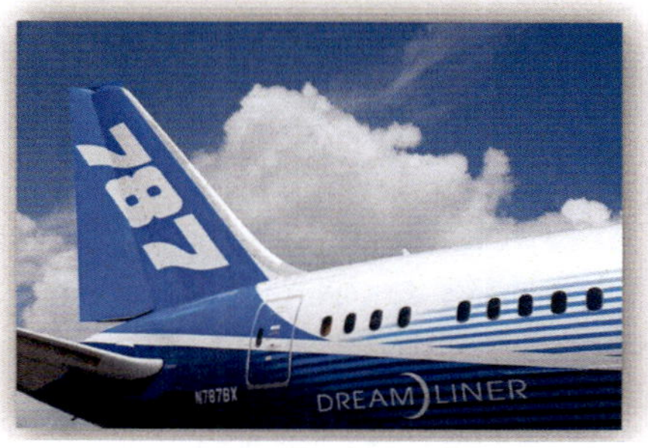

Boeing 787 Dreamliner
Thor Jorgen Udvang / Shutterstock.com

When a commercial aircraft is in-flight at a cruising altitude of 33,700 feet, the correlating outside atmospheric barometric pressure is 190 mmHg. While still flying at 33,700 feet, this same aircraft with a pressurized cabin of 7,874 feet has a modified internal barometric pressure of 577 mmHg, which in terms of O_2 concentrations is 76% of the O_2 available at sea level. The higher the barometric number in mmHg, the denser the air and the higher partial pressure of O_2. Without a pressurized cabin of around 8,000 feet, oxygen levels at 33,700 feet would be too low to sustain life, about 27% of the O_2 at sea level. Passengers

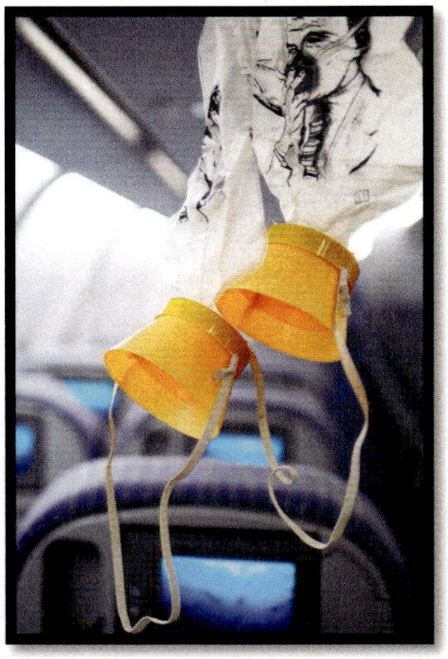

and the flight crew inside an unpressurized cabin at 33,700 feet would quickly become unconscious and would eventually die. This is the reason airlines conduct pre-flight passenger safety demonstrations involves the donning of yellow passenger O_2 masks that drop from the overhead storage bins during a rapid decompression emergency. Aircraft emergency O_2 masks at each seat deliver 10-12 minutes of O_2 when activated, just enough time for the aircraft to descend to an altitude below 12,000 feet.

6-1-4. MEDICAL COMPLICATIONS RELATED TO BEING IN-FLIGHT

The number one IFME found by Peterson et al. (2013) was syncope (fainting) followed by respiratory problems (2013). The number one medication administered for an IFME is O_2 (Rx required per FDA) (see Most Common Medications Used In-Flight). It is clear that one of the major contributors to IFMEs is the scientific fact that the majority of passengers on commercial aircraft, to some degree, suffer from mild hypoxia. The major IMFE contributors in-flight are:

- Less O_2 in the Cabin when compared to Sea Level
- 25%-30% less Partial Pressure of O_2 then at Sea Level
- Low Blood O_2 Saturation Ranges in Passengers from Between 92% and 95%
- Low Humidity in Cabin – 6% to 18%
- Dehydration
- Minimal Fresh Air
- 50% of Cabin Air Recirculated through Air Filters
- Reduced Cabin Pressure Leads to Expansion of Body Gases up to 30%
- Stationary Sitting for Long Periods (Cocks & Liew, 2007; Graf et al., 2012).

6-1-5. LOW BLOOD O_2 SATURATION IN-FLIGHT

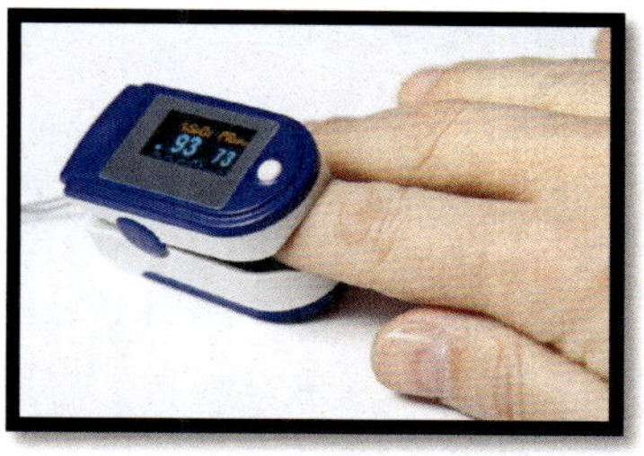

Healthy individuals at sea level should have a pulse oximeter reading of 96%-99%. When traveling by commercial airline in a pressurized cabin (pressurized to 7,874 feet), this same individual may have a pulse oximeter reading as low as 89%, but most likely between 92% and 95% (Rushkin et al., 2008).

6-1-6. IN-FLIGHT DEHYDRATION

With a humidity rate of only 6%-18%, it is quite easy for a passenger to become dehydrated within the cabin of an aircraft. Many people do not realize that moisture is withdrawn from their body with each breath they take. When combined with long flights and alcoholic beverages, a person can quickly become dehydrated. Staying hydrated in-flight can prevent many IFMEs.

6-2. ENDOTRACHEAL TUBE COMPLICATIONS AT ALTITUDE

When in-flight, air bladders expand during ascent and contract on descent. For example, a sealed bag of potato chips at sea level should be slightly inflated with air, but while in-flight, this same bag can inflate (puff-up) like a balloon to the point it pops. One of the challenges regarding in-flight medical care involves the changing pressures inside the cabin of an aircraft, which by default, affects the passengers as well.

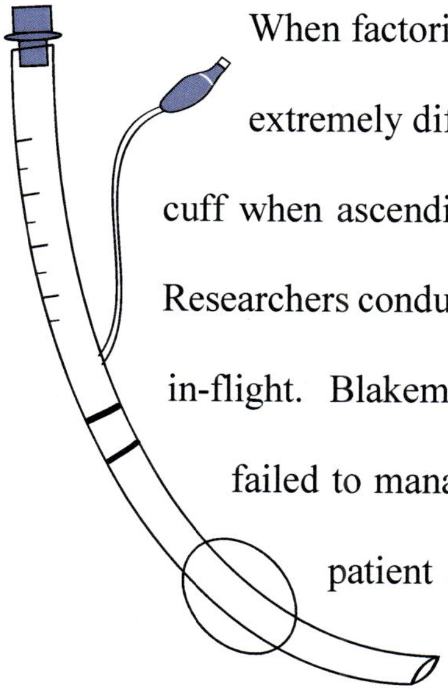

When factoring the use of the Endotracheal tube (ETT) in-flight, it has been proven to be extremely difficult to maintain the correct recommended mmHg pressure of the inflatable cuff when ascending from sea level and descending from 8,000 feet (Blakema et al., 2014). Researchers conducted a study to determine which method was most effective for using the ETT in-flight. Blakema et al. (2014) concluded that all three methods in their in-flight field tests failed to manage proper cuff pressures to avoid tracheal damage at altitude or to prevent patient aspiration of secretion's during decent. It was recommended that new techniques be developed for in-flight EET applications.

Table 8 provides the in-flight results pertaining to an 8.0 mm ETT cuff inflation control study from sea level ascending to 8,000 feet and then descending back to sea level.

Changes in Manual ETT Cuff Pressure During In-Flight Study			
	Sea Level Baseline	**8,000 Feet**	**Sea Level (after flight)**
Manual Control of ETT	**20 mmHg**	**84 mmHg**	**4 mmHg**

Table 8, Changes in ETT Cuff Pressure during In-Flight Study, Source: Blakema et al., 2014

As shown by Blakema et al., the manual ETT cuff pressure inconsistencies during the flight would have resulted in unsatisfactory conditions for the patient which may have caused further injury. The ETT cuff was only at 4 mmHg upon landing due to the cuff's stretching at 8,000 feet. Unless used at a cruising altitude with no possibility of ascent or descent cabin pressures, off-duty EMS professionals should attempt other methods of securing an airway before attempting the use of an ETT. Contact a MedLink physician for further ETT consultation.

Chapter Notes

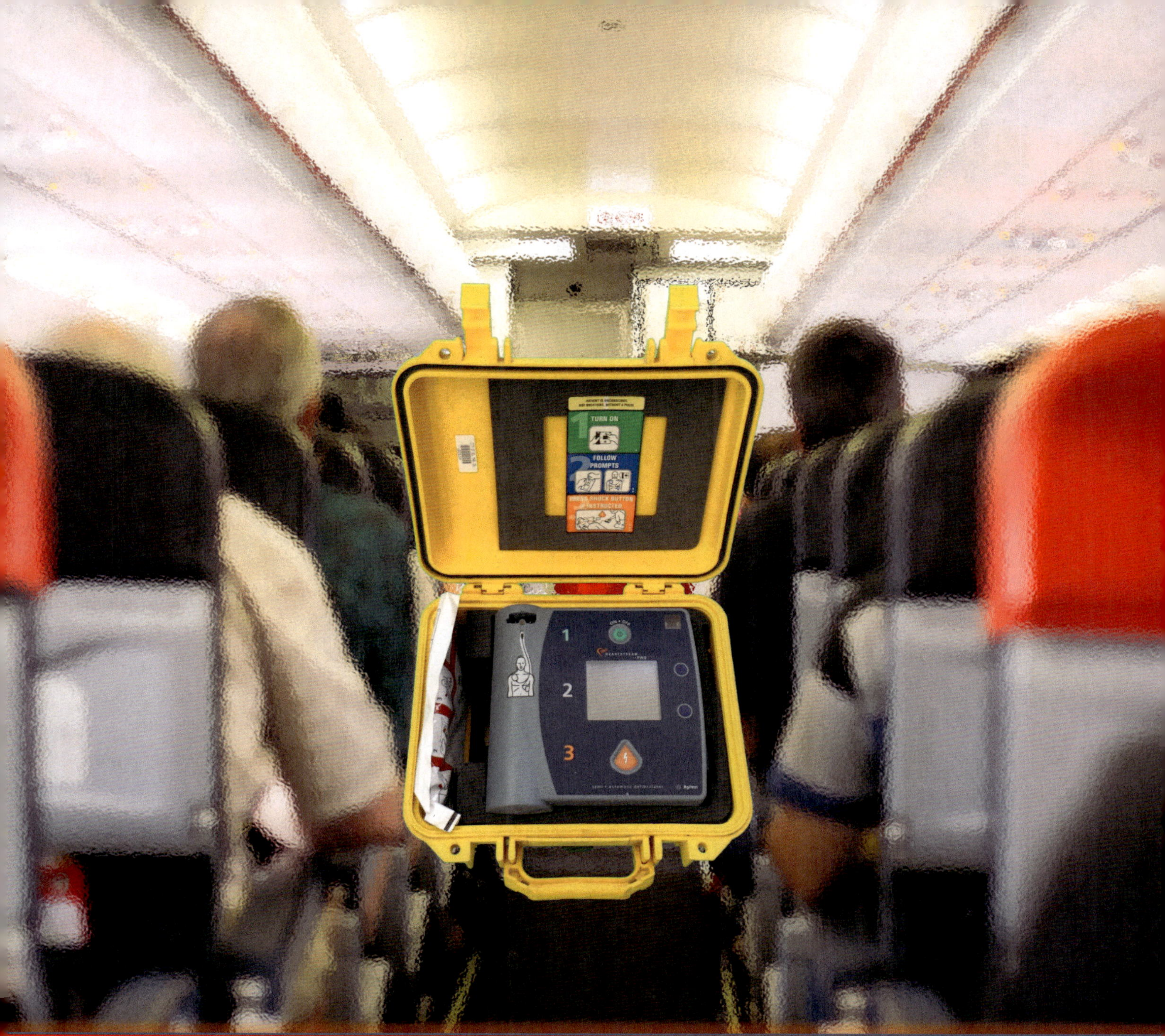

Chapter 7

Automated External Defibrillator

CHAPTER 7: HIGHLIGHTS – AUTOMATED EXTERNAL DEFIBRILLATORS

- **History of In-Flight Cardiac Arrest**
- **FAA Regulations Mandating Automated External Defibrillators (AEDs)**
  - ☑ AEDs Required on Certain Commercial Aircraft
- **Types of Defibrillators on Commercial Aircraft**
  - ☑ AEDs without EKG display
  - ☑ AEDs with EKG Display
    - EKG Monitoring Module
  - ☑ Battery Requirements
- **Telemedicine Options**

THE SURVIVAL CHAIN

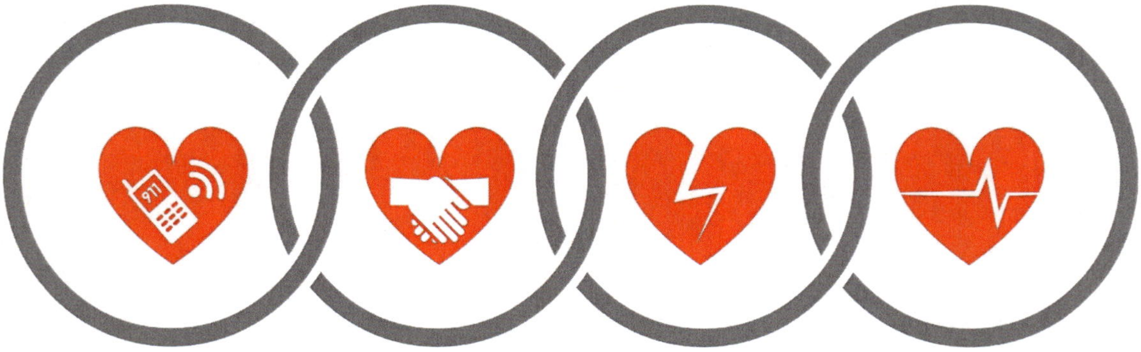

EARLY ACCESS | EARLY CPR | EARLY DEFIBRILLATION | EARLY ADVANCED CARE

7-1. HISTORY OF IN-FLIGHT CARDIAC ARREST

It is estimated that worldwide, 1000 passengers die annually while on-board commercial aircraft, mostly from a fatal heart condition known as ventricular fibrillation (VF), or cardiac arrest (O'Rourke, Donaldson, & Geddes, 1997). In many cases, a passenger who experiences sudden VF or cardiac arrest has had no prior warning signs. When VF occurs, cardiopulmonary resuscitation (CPR) is not normally adequate in reversing VF, but rather extends the time before permanent brain damage occurs and for the arrival of advanced life support (ALS). VF is treatable when immediate electrical defibrillation is applied to the patient. In terms of survivability, "VF is critically dependent on the time of onset to the first defibrillatory shock" (O'Rourke, Donaldson, & Geddes, 1997, p. 2850); shocks applied within 3 minutes of onset have the highest probability of survival. The question of diverting an aircraft for ALS ground care for a passenger suffering from cardiac arrest, even with high quality CPR is not a viable alternative to the in-flight defibrillator. If a patient in VF is delayed a defibrillator shock beyond 16 minutes, the patient will generally not survive (O'Rourke, Donaldson, & Geddes, 1997). Beginning as early as 1991, airlines began experimenting with the idea of carrying automated external defibrillators on aircraft. After initial tests and trials, several airlines began training crewmembers on the use of AEDs on designated international fights well before regulation required them. Initial results looked promising. Over a 65-month study period, Qantas airlines reported out of six incidents of witnessed cardiac arrest, five were converted to a purposeful heart rhythm (one remained in VF) which resulted in the long-term survival of two of these patients (O'Rourke, Donaldson, & Geddes, 1997).

Page et al. (2000) conducted a study of 200 incidents regarding AED deployments with American Airlines (between 1997 and 1999) and the study concluded that AED use was "effective, with an excellent rate of survival" (p. 1210), 40% of those shocked with an AED were eventually discharged from the hospital. The authors of this study also concluded that out of 13 viable patients in VF, the AEDs sensitivity was 100% on target and indicated to deliver a shock, with the first shock in all cases terminating the VF. Interestingly, in over 50% of the AED deployments on commercial aircraft, the AEDs were not being used to defibrillate patients. The AEDs were being used to monitor heart rhythms of conscious patients who were generally suffering from cardiac complications. It is generally not advised to attach AED shock pads to a conscious passenger unless the AED specifically has a monitor mode.

7-2. FAA REGULATIONS MANDATING AUTOMATED EXTERNAL DEFIBRILLATORS

With new data showing the importance of AEDs on-board commercial aircraft, in 1998 the FAA began requiring the training and use of AEDs on commercial aircraft (Federal Aviation Administration, 2006). FAA regulation requires that AEDs used on commercial aircraft must be approved for medical use by the U.S. Food and Drug Administration (FDA) and their batteries must be approved for aircraft use (Federal Aviation Administration, 2006).

Continue to Next Page

7-2-1. FAA REGULATION CFR 121.803(C) (4) REQUIRING AUTOMATED EXTERNAL DEFIBRILLATORS

The FAA regulation requiring AEDs on aircraft has been amended since the law was written in 1998. The current version of the regulation is cited below:

> *CFR 121.803*
>
> *(c) For treatment of injuries, medical events, or minor accidents that might occur during flight time each airplane must have the following equipment that meets the specifications and requirements of appendix A of this part:*
>
> *(4) In airplanes for which a flight attendant is required and with a maximum payload capacity of more than 7,500 pounds, an approved automated external defibrillator as of April 12, 2004. (U.S. Government Publishing Office, 2015b).*

7-2-2. DEFIBRILLATOR SAFETY PRECAUTIONS

While the FAA and ESAS do not require a specific manufacturer of an AED on commercial aircraft, there are a couple of safety requirements pertaining to the use of the AED:

- ☑ The AED must be approved for medical use by the FDA
- ☑ The AED should be equipped with a battery designed for aircraft use
- ☑ The AED shall not deliver a shock to a patient within 10 feet of an open oxygen source

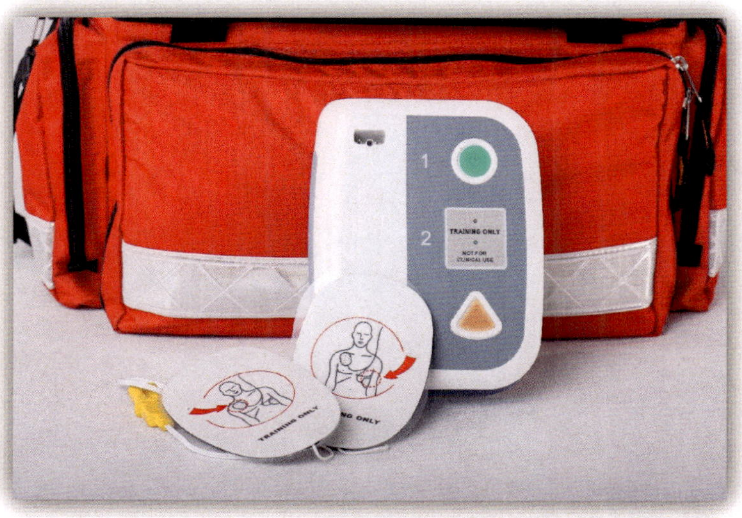

7-3. TYPES OF DEFIBRILLATORS ON COMMERCIAL AIRCRAFT

When referring to commercial airline AEDs, there are generally two types of models (with and without displays) as shown below with the Phillips Hearth Start FR2+ and the Cardiac Science Powerheart G3.

1) AED with a EKG display

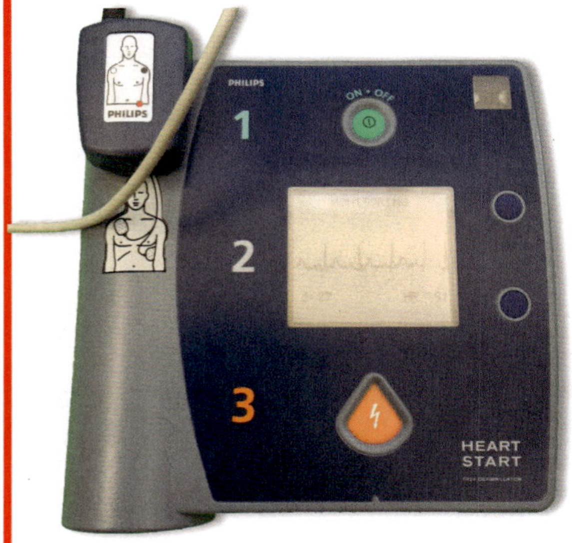

2) AED with no EKG display

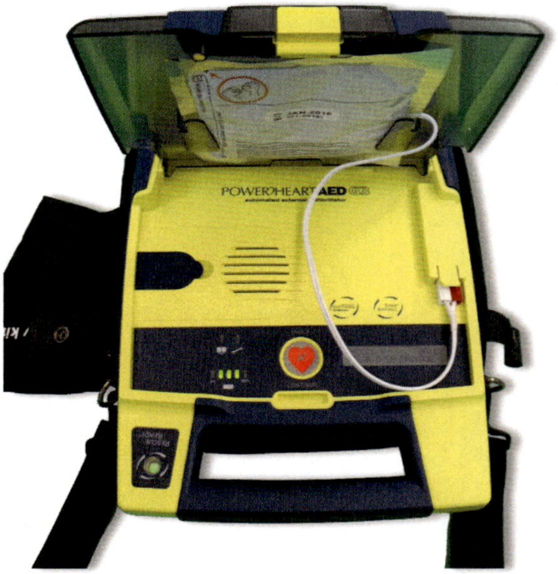

7-3-1. AUTOMATED EXTERNAL DEFIBRILLATOR WITH NO DISPLAY

In terms of automatically interpreting a shockable rhythm such as VF on a patient and delivering a shock, there is no difference between an AED with or without a display, they will both function in a similar manner. Both models have a voice prompt that will read aloud instructions such as the following:

1) Plug in pads connector
2) Place pads against bare chest
3) Analyzing - stand back - do not touch the patient
4) Shock advised – charging – do not touch the patient
5) Press flashing button to shock patient
6) Shock delivered

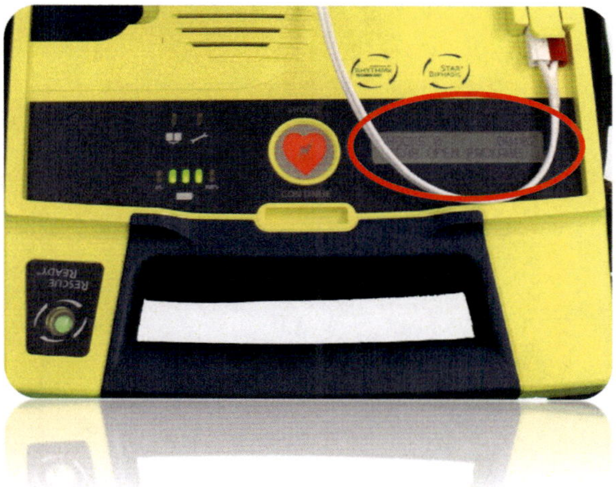

Note: If a user cannot hear the voice prompts due to noise, there may be a small character display with instructions on the AED. If users are not familiar with the in-flight AED – they should ask a crewmember for help, all flight attendants are required to be AED trained and certified.

7-3-2. AED WITH EKG DISPLAY

The primary difference between AEDs with or without a display is the fact that the heart rhythm is visible in real time with the display models. This can be extremely important when treating and monitoring a patient suffering from heart complications. Some AEDs have add-on heart monitor attachments:

- The Phillips FR2+ has an additional component called the "EKG module" which turns the AED into a heart monitor.
- The Phillips EKG module makes it impossible to shock a patient when in monitoring mode.
- If a shock-able rhythm is detected with the EKG module, the AED would notify the user with voice prompts to remove the module and plug in pads to analyze.
- The EKG module is an important safety component when only monitoring is desired.

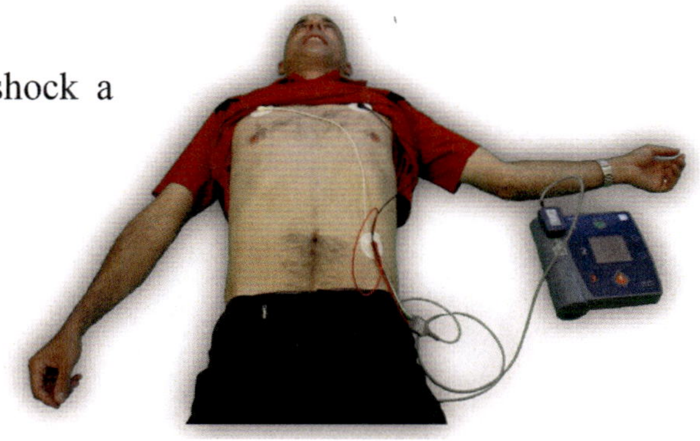

Phillips FR2+ with EKG Module

From past data collected from various AED studies, it appears that most AEDs carried aboard commercial aircraft have been equipped with an Electrocardiogram (ECG or EKG) display. The Page et al. (2000) study reported that 50.5% of the 200 AED applications were administered to conscious patients who reported chest pain and/or discomfort. The Peterson et al. (2013) study reported similar results.

7-3-2-1. AED Picture with EKG Monitoring Module

3- Lead EKG Module

- Phillips FR2+ AED with attached 3-lead EKG module
- EKG monitor mode only
- No voice prompts
- Will not analyze or shock patient
- Safe for conscious patients

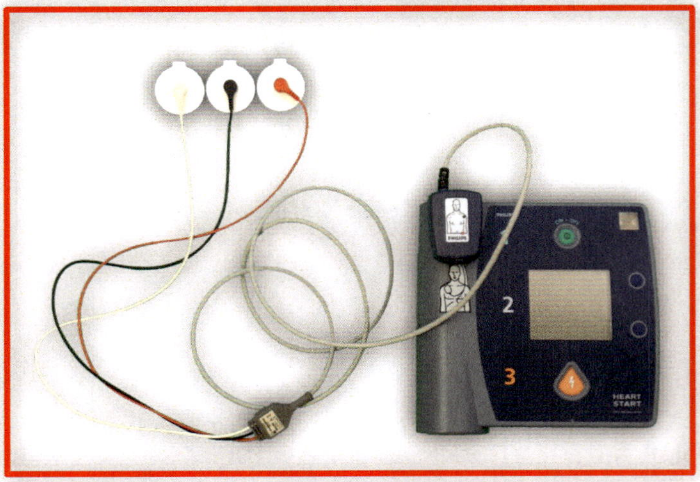

7-3-3. AED PICTURE WITH DEFIBRILLATOR PADS

Defibrillator Pads

- Phillips FR2+ AED with attached Defibrillator Pads
- Designed to be used on an unresponsive patient in cardiac arrest - VF
- Pads will analyze and shock
- Pads will continue to monitor EKG once initiated
- Will advise to analyze every two minutes or instruct to continue CPR

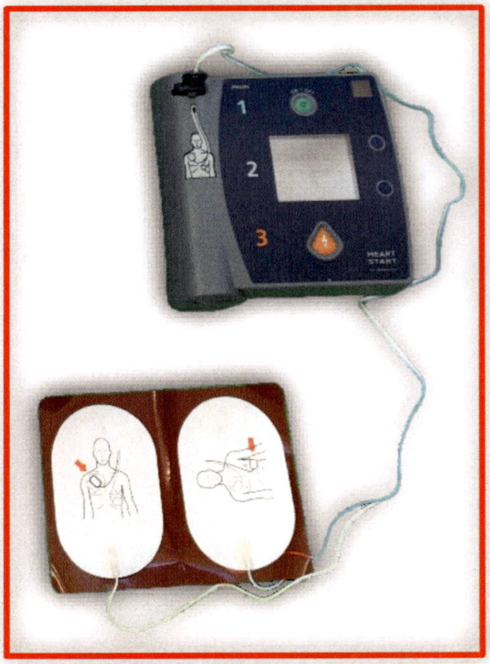

7-3-4. AED BATTERY REQUIREMENTS

After April 30, 2005, all commercial aircraft that are required to carry an AED on-board, must ensure that the AEDs in service have an approved battery or power source that meets FAA Technical Standard Order requirements for electronic devices used in aviation (U.S. Government Publishing Office, 2015d). Most AED batteries are rechargeable or non-rechargeable lithium-ion types.

7-4. TELEMEDICINE OPTIONS

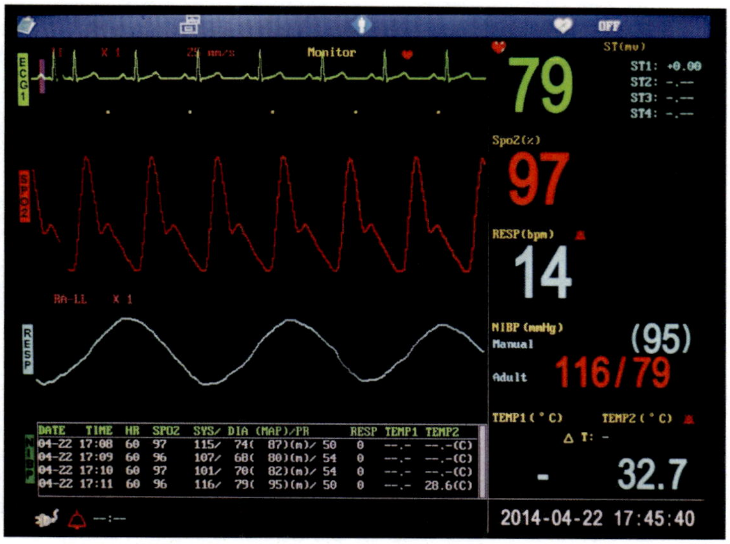

Only a handful of European Union airlines carry telemedicine devices such as the RDTs Tempus IC vital signs monitor (sold by MedAire) aboard their aircraft. The RDT Tempus IC vital signs monitor is essentially a sophisticated ALS monitor that has fully integrated medical parameters, voice and video conferencing, a satellite/radio transmitter, and can allow an untrained passenger to collect and transmit vital sign data to MedLink physicians on the ground (Campbell, 2007). Airlines with telemedicine monitors allow MedLink physicians to get real time vital signs and medical data that would otherwise be impossible without on-board off-duty EMS professionals. The RDT Tempus IC can identify and transmit indicators of medical severity to ground-based physicians regarding the patient's health status and either recommend diversion or continuation of the flight.

Dr. Alves reiterated that the decision to divert an aircraft is complex. Whenever MedLink physicians can get real-time medical data, it benefits both the patient and the airline to ensure the correct decisions are made in-flight regarding treatment and whether the flight needs to be diverted.

Chapter Notes

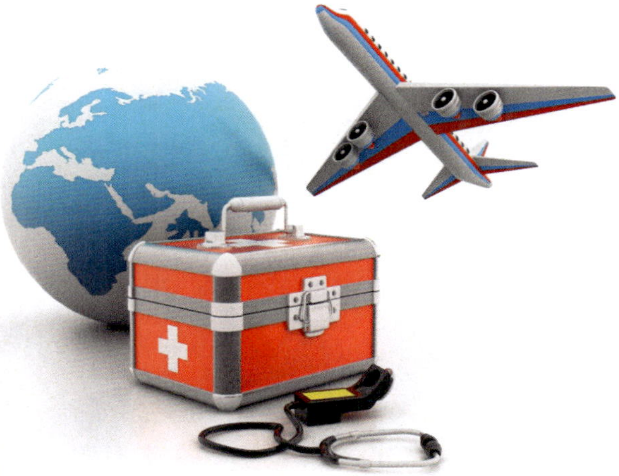

Chapter 8

In-Flight Medical Emergencies

TOP 10

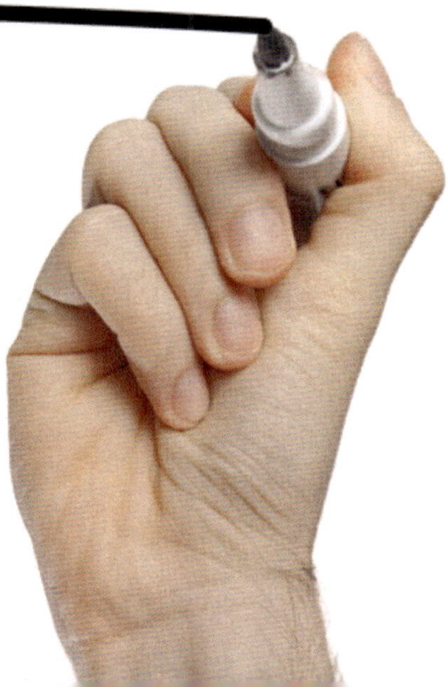

By Category

CHAPTER 8: HIGHLIGHTS – TOP 10 IN-FLIGHT MEDICAL EMERGENCIES

- **Only 17% of All IFMEs Are Reported Worldwide**
  - ☑ Not Every In-Flight Medical Emergency is Recorded
  - ☑ No Current Regulations that Require Airlines to Report IFMEs
  - ☑ Patients and Hospitals Do Not Inform Airlines of Patient Diagnosis/Outcomes
- **List - Top 10 IFMEs**
- **The Only Reportable Medical Incidents Required by the FAA are In-Flight Deaths**
  - ☑ Deaths Occur Very Rarely In-Flight (0.3% To 1.3% of Estimated IFMEs)
- **Current Data Reported on IFMEs is Not Very Reliable**
  - ☑ No Global IFME Registry
  - ☑ Some Reports Indicate Cardiac as #1 Medical Problem, Others - Syncope as #1, and Others - Neurological (Stroke) as #1
  - ☑ Need for IFME Registry to be Developed by FAA / EASA

8-1. NO AIRLINE STANDARD FOR COLLECTING IN-FLIGHT MEDICAL EMERGENCY DATA

Accurate calculations regarding the number of IFMEs on airlines has always been difficult, primarily because they are not required to report these events (Silverman & Gendreau, 2008). It is estimated that only 17% of the IFMEs that occur worldwide are reported, and of those reported, most resulted in hospitalization and/or death of the passenger. The other problem with tracking IFME data is that most U.S. registered airlines fly internationally, not just domestically. Each country is responsible for creating its own IFME tracking program if it chooses to do so. The only method currently used for reporting IFMEs is from scarce and unreliable data. This data suggests approximately 50-100 IFMEs occur per day on U.S. registered commercial airlines. An IFME study from one airline found that one out of every 11,000 passengers experienced an IFME (Buchanan et al., 2014). When airline passengers are admitted to local hospitals, the airlines rarely find out the prognosis or outcome of the passenger due to privacy laws. In the U. S., the only reliable data pertaining to IFMEs is when there is a death related to the event, which is very rare at approximately 0.3%.

Continue to Next Page

8-2. TOP 10 LIST OF IFMES

Top 10 In-Flight Medical Emergencies by Symptom

Percentages in **bold and underlined** represent #1 percentage in category

Number	Symptom (Chief Complaint)	Percentage	Aircraft Diversion	Transported to ER	Admitted to Hospital
1	Syncope	**<u>37.4%</u>**	5%	22.1%	6.5%
2	Respiratory Symptoms	12.1%	5.6%	22.7%	10.6%
3	Nausea / Vomiting	9.5%	4.9%	23.7%	6.1%
4	Cardiac Symptoms	7.7%	**<u>18.4%</u>**	**<u>45.5%</u>**	21%
5	Seizures	5.8%	12%	35.8%	12.5%
6	Abdominal Pain	4.1%	10.2%	39.8%	10.5%
7	Infectious Disease	2.8%	1.8%	18.8%	3.4%
8	Agitation and/or Psychiatric symptoms	2.4%	5.6%	15.3%	7%
9	Allergic Reaction	2.2%	4.5%	17.2%	3.5%
10	CVA / Stroke	2%	16.4%	43%	**<u>23.3%</u>**

This chart is based on data from call records to the STAT-MD ground-based physician communications center involving five domestic and international airlines from January 1, 2008, through October 31, 2010 (Peterson et al., 2013, p. 2077).

Note: Because this data was provided by a ground-based physician call center (STAT-MD) and not the airlines, these IFMEs were severe enough to warrant the activation of this service which does not represent the true or total number of IFMEs over this study period. According to Dr. Alves (2015), many airlines in the United States call MedLink as a last resort during IFMEs and not as a common practice.

8-2-1. REVIEW OF THE TOP 10 IN-FLIGHT MEDICAL EMERGENCIES LIST

Syncope (fainting), was rated as the number one IFME chief complaint during the Peterson et al. (2013) study which resulted in a 5% diversion rate with 22.1% of the patients being transported to local hospitals. Cardiac symptoms, which was listed as number four on the list, represented the greatest number of flight diversions (18.4%) and the greatest number of patients being transported to local hospitals (45.5%). Interestingly, the last on the list at number 10, cerebral vascular accident (CVA) and stroke, represented only (2%) of the total IFMEs but resulted in the second greatest number of diversions (16.4%) and the greatest number of patient hospital admissions (23.3%).

8-3. REPORTABLE MEDICAL INCIDENTS REQUIRED BY THE FAA INCLUDE ALL IN-FLIGHT DEATHS

All in-flight related deaths occurring on United States registered aircraft must be reported to the FAA or the National Transportation Safety Board (NTSB) (see: 10-4 - Airlines are Required to Report In-Flight Deaths).

8-3-1. DEATHS OCCUR VERY RARELY IN-FLIGHT

Current data reported on IFMEs is not very reliable. The slivers of data that we do have suggests that in-flights deaths are extremely low. The Peterson et al., (2013) study found that the death rate was 0.3% among all patients involved with an IFME. This same study indicated that a previous study found death rates were between 0.3% and 1.3% of all IFMEs. O'Rourke et al., (1997) estimate that approximately 1,000 passengers die on commercial airlines each year. Since official numbers of IFMEs do not exist, one can only speculate and make an educated guess. There currently is no global registry for IFMEs and until that happens, it will remain difficult to determine the actual numbers of both IFMEs and the resulting deaths that occur in-flight.

Chapter Notes

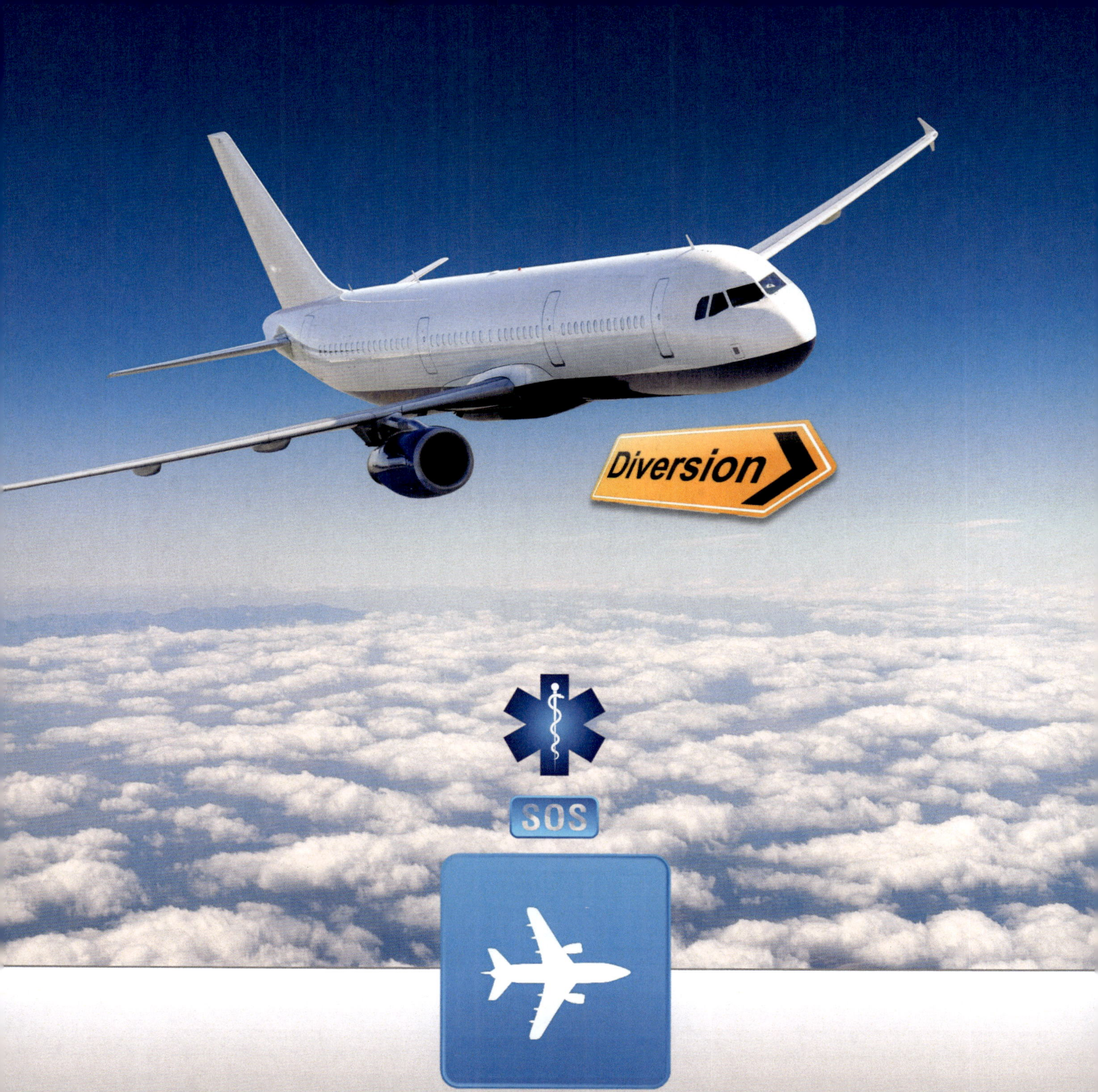

Chapter 9

Diversion of Aircraft

CHAPTER 9: HIGHLIGHTS – DIVERSION OF AIRCRAFT

- **Data Related to Diversions**
  - ☑ List of Most Common IFME Diversions
  - ☑ Diversion Benefits and Complications
    - Aircraft Diversion when No Medical Help Available On-Board
    - Aircraft Diversion for the Safety of the Passengers
    - Diversion of Aircraft for a Deceased Passenger
- **Considerations and Perspectives on when to Divert Flight**
  - ☑ Pilot's Decision to Divert Based on Several Factors
  - ☑ MedLink or Off-Duty EMS Professional's Recommendation
- **Costs to Airline and Passengers to Divert an Aircraft**
  - ☑ Emergency Fuel Dump and Fuel Costs
  - ☑ Ticket Refunds
  - ☑ Trip Insurance Claims
  - ☑ Lodging and Meals
  - ☑ Delays and Lost Work

9-1. DATA RELATED TO DIVERSIONS

Data indicates there are more reported occurrences of IFMEs on long-haul flights when compared to short-leg commuter flights, this is primarily due to the duration of time spent on the aircraft (Peterson et al., 2013). Captain Ian Stocke, a U.S. commuter airlines pilot corroborated this data indicating that under his watch, IFMEs were extremely rare. Duration of the flight and the number of passengers on board are generally the two key factors in predicting the likelihood of an IFME. When attempting to predict the likelihood of an IFME aircraft diversion, one should consider: 1) type of medical emergency, 2) type of medical professionals available to assist, 3) location of aircraft (domestic or international), 4) the size of aircraft, 5) and the fight duration. The likelihood of an IFME occurring are as follows:

- Odds of an IFME on all U.S. commercial airlines (30 to 300 passengers) - 1 in 604 flights
- Odds of an IFME on International Jumbo Jets (400+ passengers) – 1 in 26 flight

(Graf et al., 2012; NOAA, 2015; Peterson et al., 2013)

In reference to the above data, it appears that a great predictor of the likelihood of an IFME is the number of passengers on-board an aircraft. The larger the aircraft as measured by the seats on-board, the greater the likelihood of an IFME, which also increases the likelihood of a medical related diversion of the aircraft. In relation to all airline flights, long-haul international flights with 400+ passengers are 25 times more likely to experience an IFME, which increases the chance of diversion. To further complicate the prediction of medically related diversions on commercial airlines, the new generations of jumbo jets such as the Airbus A380-900 and Boeing 777-200/300 fly further and carry more passengers than previous wide-body aircraft. As an example, the A380-900 has a manufacture's estimated range of 8,200 nautical miles, a fight endurance of 18 hours, and a maximum passenger capability of 853 passengers (Airbus, 2015; Sand et al., 2012; Silverman & Gendreau, 2008). Aircraft like the Airbus A380-900 will, without a doubt, increase the odds of an IFME by another 200% when compared to a 400 passenger Boeing 747. This equates to an IFME on these jumbo aircraft every 12-14 flights, meaning more flight delays due to diversions for medical emergencies. Airlines operating these new generation jumbo jets may have to consider hiring medical crew members or implementing new fly miles "Doctors & EMTs On-Board" programs to ensure passengers are well cared for in-flight.

Data does indicates that the even on critical IFMEs such as with cardiac arrest, 42% of these incidents are not diverted because the aircraft is unable to divert (e.g. flight over the ocean) (Peterson et al., 2013). In another study involving the STAT-MD call center, only 7.3% of IFME calls ended in diversion (University of Pittsburgh, 2013).

9-1-1. LIST OF THE MOST COMMON IFME DIVERSIONS

Certain medical emergencies have a higher occurrence of diversions, especially on international flights. These IFMEs would include:

- ✓ Cardiac 26.4% (chest pain most common)
- ✓ Neurological 19.5% (stroke most common)
- ✓ Gastrointestinal 11.4%
- ✓ Syncope 10% (Rahim Valani, 2010) (See: 2-4-2 - Diversion of Aircraft)

9-1-2. DIVERSION BENEFITS AND COMPLICATIONS

Diversion of a commercial aircraft most often has the greatest impact on the ill passenger and in many cases, may mean the difference between life and death. When time is of the essence, especially with neurological and cardiac complications, the earlier the patient receives medical care inside a hospital, the better their prognosis. When a stroke or CVA occurs in-flight, the passenger needs not just a hospital, but an available stroke center that specializes in emergency medical treatment of CVAs. If a CVA patient reaches a stroke center within one hour of onset, they will have the best chances of survival with the least neurological side effects. For this reason, the majority of CVA cases will result in diversion of the aircraft if the plane is not already preparing to land.

9-1-2-1. Aircraft Diverson when No Medical Help On-Board

When IFMEs occur and no medical help is available on-board the aircraft, flight diversion may be warranted and the flight crew should contact MedLink or similar service for guidance.

9-1-2-2. Aircraft Diversion for the Safety of the Passengers

Another reason diversion may be the correct option is when the passengers in the cabin are under duress and/or in fear of their safety. There have been documented cases of agitated passengers acting bizarrely, and even trying to attack the flight crew and thier passengers. In 1999, a male passenger aboard a Hungarian National Airlines flight attacked the captain, crew, and the passengers (tried to light a woman's hair on fire) and was ultimately sedated and restrained (Kovac, 1999) (See: 3-1-2 Captain Can Overrule the Recommendations of a Medical Professional). The male passenger ended up dying as a result of his medical emergency. Law enforcement describe this agitated behavior as excited delirium syndrome (ExDS), a "serious and potentially deadly medical condition involving psychotic behavior, elevated temperature, and an extreme fight-or-flight response by the nervous system. Failure to recognize the symptoms and involve emergency medical services (EMS) to provide appropriate medical treatment may lead to death" (Roach et al., 2014, para 1).

9-1-2-3. Diversion of Aircraft for a Deceased Passenger

Lufthansa Airlines believes that if there is no other immediate emergency related to the death of a passenger, there would be no valid reason to divert the aircraft. Lufthansa states:

> "The affected person cannot be helped any further, and an unplanned landing would only create problems with the relatives of the deceased and the other passengers: decontamination and quarantine regulations, undetermined causes of death with potential legal consequences and subsequent transport of the corpse back home" (Gabel et al., 2011, p. 137).

Each airline will have their own policies regarding flight diversions for deceased passengers and some airlines may decide to divert for a death on-board regardless of the consequences to the passengers.

9-2. CONSIDERATIONS AND PERSPECTIVES ON WHEN TO DIVERT FLIGHT

When the captain of an aircraft is asked to divert a flight to a closer airport, there are several factors to consider. Not all of the factors are about the ill passenger's fate either. The safety of the aircraft and all those on-board must be factored into the decision to divert an aircraft. The following list includes examples of what a flight crew must consider before diverting to a closer airport:

- ✈Condition of the ill passenger
- ✈Is the passenger stable
- ✈Ability of off-duty EMS to handle IFME
- ✈MedLink physician recommendation
- ✈Off-duty EMS professional recommendation
- ✈Equipment needed (e.g. ventilator, surgical)
- ✈CPR & CVA are the most diverted IFMEs
- ✈Urgent indication for immediate hospitalization
- ✈Distance to next suitable runway with medical facilities, EMS
- ✈Airport services (e.g. refueling, terminals, food, hotels)
- ✈Weight of aircraft upon landing (need to dump fuel)
- ✈Pilot preparations to divert (30 minutes)
- ✈Regulatory requirements of crew (e.g. need new pilots and crew to continue flight once landed) (Gabel, et al., 2011).

9-2-1. CAPTAIN'S DECISION TO DIVERT BASED ON SEVERAL FACTORS

The captain of an aircraft will listen to the recommendations from the flight attendants, the off-duty EMS professional, and the ground-based physician to determine if diverting the aircraft would be the best decision for the current circumstances. The MedLink ground-based physician service has a database of thousands of medical facilities located all over the world. For a diversion to be done successfully, the aircraft has to be diverted to an airport that has accessible nearby medical facilities to handle the specific medical emergency in question. The facility must also have available medical staff to accept an incoming patient. MedLink will make all the arrangements with the airports, hospitals, and ground-based EMS personnel to help the captain of the aircraft make a well, informed decision of whether or not to divert. For this reason, if there is a dispute between the off-duty EMS professional and the MedLink physician, the captain of the aircraft will usually choose to comply with the advice from the MedLink physician (Rushkin et al., 2008)

9-2-2. DIVERTING A COMMUTER AIRCRAFT

When an IFME is presented to the crew and no off-duty EMS professionals are available, Captain Stocke explained that his priority is to divert the aircraft to the closest airport to ensure the passenger receives the best medical care possible. Even when off-duty EMS professionals are available to help, in most cases commuter flights will be diverted to closer airports due to the lack of potential treatment locations on-board.

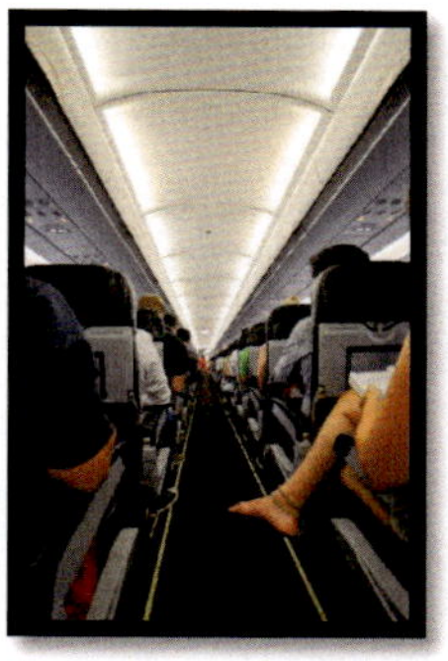

Combined with the lack of open space, a very narrow aisle, and only one or two flight attendants on-board, caring for an ill passenger on a commuter aircraft is challenging and dangerous. Due to these reasons, commuter pilots are generally more inclined to divert to a closer airport for ground-based EMS (Stocke, 2015).

9-3. COSTS TO AIRLINE AND PASSENGERS TO DIVERT AN AIRCRAFT

Due to many unknown costs at the time of an emergency, commercial airline flight diversions related to IFMEs can range from $15,000 to $893,000 (Rushkin et al., 2008). These costs may include fuel that was dumped for landing, hotels, food, passenger delays, replacement crews, change in aircraft, lost work, travel insurance, and ticket refunds. In regards to a deceased passenger on an international flight, it is generally easier on both the airline and the family members, when a flight in this situation continues to its original destination. It may be extremely costly for a family to fly the deceased home from a foreign country.

Chapter Notes

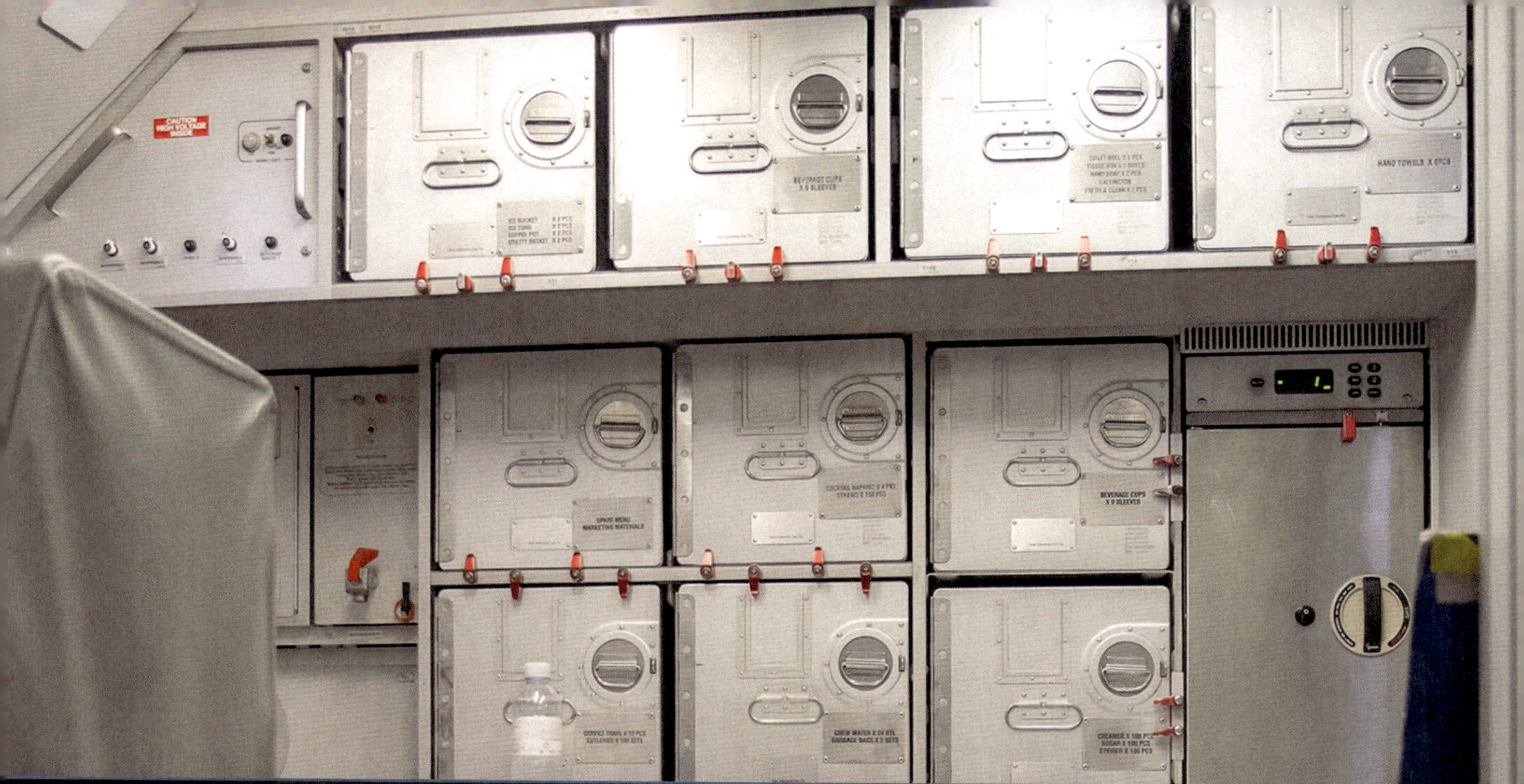

Chapter 10

Death of Passenger In-Flight

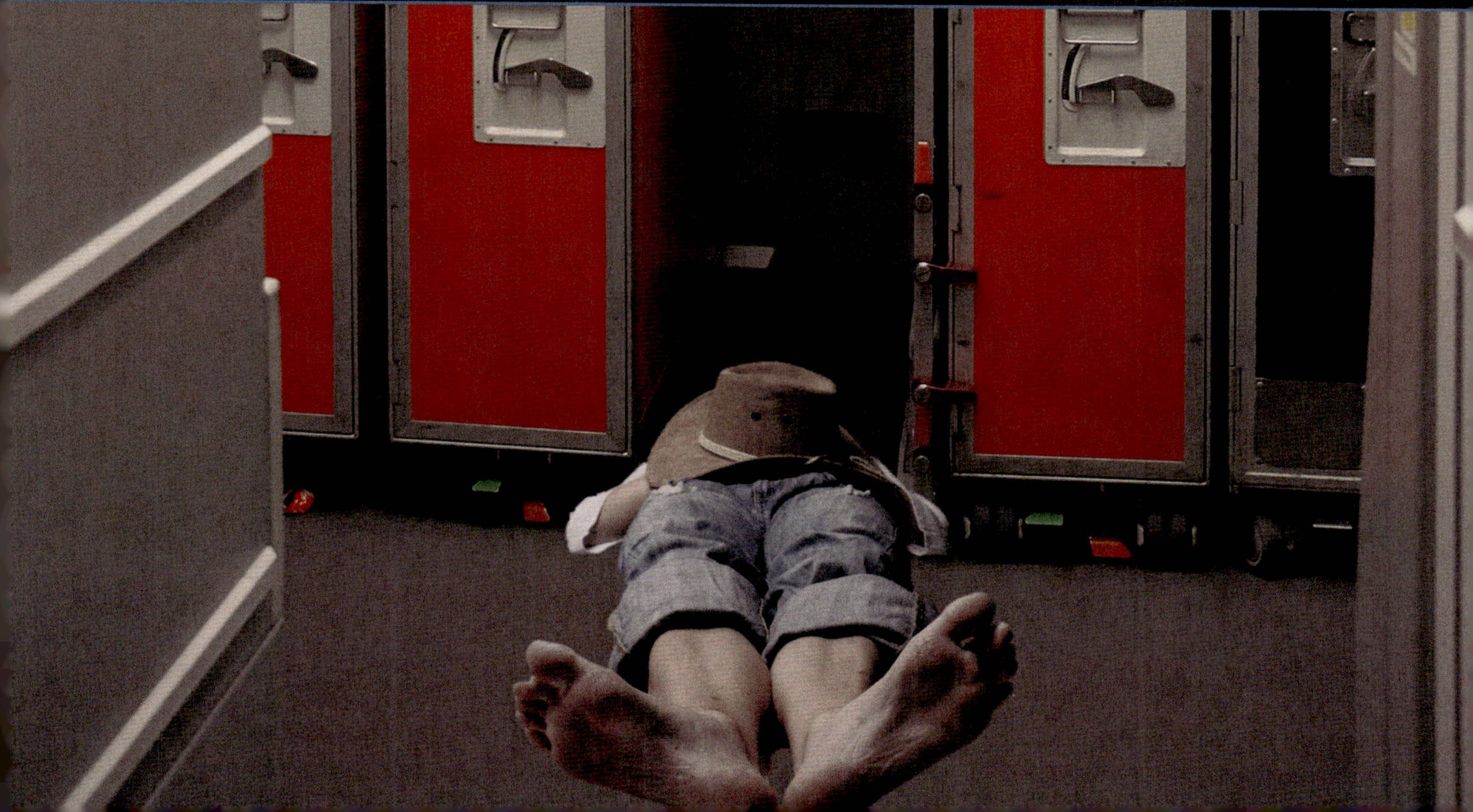

CHAPTER 10: HIGHLIGHTS – DEATH OF PASSENGER IN-FLIGHT

- **Off-Duty EMS – Handling the Death of a Passenger**
    - ☑ Two Types of In-Flight Death Scenarios
        - Found Dead
        - Witnessed Medical Distress – Resuscitation Unsuccessful
- **Locations on Plane for Resuscitation Efforts or Storage of Deceased**
    - ☑ Galley Areas Shall Be Used for Treatment of Patient and/or Storage of Body
        - Attempt to Resuscitate for at Least 30 Minutes Prior to Presuming Dead
        - Do Not Resuscitate (DNR) Order
- **Presumption of Death In-Flight**
- **Storage of a Body In-Flight**
    - ☑ Storage of Body
    - ☑ Airline In-Flight Death Policies
    - ☑ Divert when Safe for Aircraft and Passengers
    - ☑ Be Truthful when Asked Questions by Other Passengers
    - ☑ Do Not Store Body Next to Unaware Passengers
- **Airlines Requirement to Report Death**
    - ☑ Must Advise Local Authorities of In-Flight Death
    - ☑ Must Report In-Flight Accidents / Injuries to NTSB

10-1. OFF-DUTY EMS – HANDLING THE DEATH OF A PASSENGER

Off-duty EMS professionals shall refer to the airline crew for the handling of an in-flight death. If the crew members do not take an immediate and/or an appropriate role in the handling of an in-flight death, this chapter will provide peer-reviewed best practices for the handling of an in-flight death.

10-1-1. TWO TYPES OF DEATH SCENARIOS

Although there may be several ways a person may die during a commercial aircraft flight, in terms of this manual, there are two possibilities. The passenger was either found dead (unable to wake up the passenger) or the passenger was observed to be in medical distress and resuscitation efforts were unsuccessful.

10-1-1-1. Found Dead

Passengers may be found dead from presumed natural causes while sitting in his/her assigned seat or even in the lavatory. Typically, a deceased passenger would be found after a night flight or during a cabin service (Gabel, et al., 2011). Once it is determined that the passenger is dead from obvious signs of death, the best option would be to store the body in a manner consistent with the airline's policy related to in-flight deaths.

10-1-1-2. Unsuccessful Resuscitation Efforts

When a passenger has been observed with symptoms of sudden medical distress or cardiac arrest, every effort shall be made to provide immediate medical care to assist that passenger, including CPR and the application of an AED. If efforts to resuscitate the passenger are unsuccessful (no signs of life) for a period of at least 30 minutes, medical care may cease and the presumption of death may be made (Alves, 2015; Stone, Lubarsky, & Agarwal, 2014).

10-2. LOCATIONS ON PLANE FOR RESUSCITATION EFFORTS OR STORAGE OF DECEASED

The cabin of a commercial aircraft is cramped, loud, and at times dark. If an off-duty EMS professional is summoned to an IFME, the main factor in determining if a passenger shall be moved to a more suitable location is if the passenger is unresponsive. Not much, in terms of checking vital signs and providing lifesaving measures, can be done with a patient slumped over in their seat. The average leg space between seats in coach is measured in inches, so there is no practical way of assessing an unresponsive passenger when seated. For persons who are unresponsive, they shall be moved to a more suitable location; the aisle shall be avoided when possible on single aisle narrow-body aircraft. This can be achieved in the following manner:

- Ask nearby passengers in the same row to temporarily move out of their seats so the patient can be laid down across several seats for assessing vital signs.
- If CPR is needed, an easily accessible hard flat surface which allows for movement of multiple persons is recommended. The following areas may be utilized for an unresponsive patient:
  - ☑ The aisle on a wide-body aircraft when two aisles exist
  - ☑ Emergency exit floor space
  - ☑ Galley
  - ☑ First class cabin
  - ☑ Crew stations

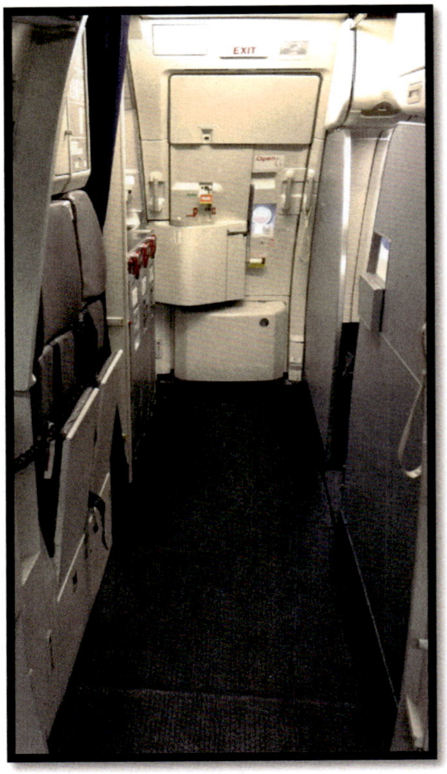

Front Galley / Boarding Door on an Airbus A319

10-2-1. GALLEY AREAS SHALL BE USED FOR TREATMENT OF PATIENT AND/OR STORAGE OF BODY

Even on small aircraft, the galley area is going to provide the largest space for the treatment and/or storage of a passenger. With larger aircraft, there will be numerous treatment/storage location options. Ideally, the passenger shall be moved to the most suitable location that is nearest to the aircraft's front passenger boarding door if resuscitation is needed and ground-based EMS are meeting the plane at the gate. Resuscitation efforts with CPR, an AED, and BVM are only possible in a large area of the aircraft where the floor is flat. It may be difficult to perform IFME assessments on smaller aircraft and in these instances, diversion to a closer airport may be warranted.

10-2-2. ATTEMPT TO RESUSCITATE FOR AT LEAST 30 MINUTES PRIOR TO PRESUMING DEAD

If CPR and resuscitation efforts of a passenger are unsuccessful in-flight, the best practice for ceasing medical assistance is provided by the International Air Transport Association (IATA). If off-duty EMS professionals are unable to regain a pulse with no shockable rhythm for 30 minutes "2012 guidelines put forth by the IATA state that in such a circumstance, the patient can be presumed dead and CPR ceased" (Stone, Lubarsky, & Agarwal, 2014, p. 131).

10-2-3. DO NOT RESUSCITATE (DNR) ORDER

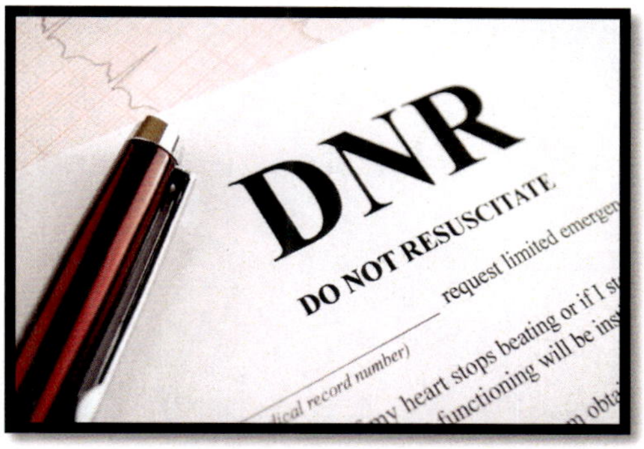

If an off-duty EMS professional is presented with a DNR order by a family member of an ill passenger, that order shall be respected if deemed authentic and properly signed. If no written DNR order is presented at the time of the IFME, off-duty EMS professionals shall continue resuscitation efforts until instructed otherwise from the crew or captain of the flight or 30 minutes of CPR have passed with no pulse or shockable rhythm.

10-3. PRESUMPTION OF DEATH IN-FLIGHT

MedAire Global Medical Director, Dr. Alves (2015), confirmed during a telephonic interview that MedLink physicians cannot pronounce a person dead in-flight and will instruct the off-duty EMS professional to make a presumption of death if the following applies:

1. If after 30 minutes of CPR, there is no shockable rhythm or signs of life.
2. If the passenger displays obvious signs of death (i.e., rigor mortis).

It shall be also noted that a physician on-board an aircraft shall not pronounce a person dead in-flight either because this can only be done in the territory of the county where the aircraft lands. When in-flight, the territory/state of where the death occurs is unknown, so the death is pronounced when the plane lands in accordance with local regulations.

10-3-1. WHERE SHOULD THE CABIN CREW STORE A BODY IN-FLIGHT

When previous deaths have occurred in-flight, there have been reports of horrified passengers who have woken up to a dead corpse in the seat next to them. In 2007, this is exactly what happened to British Airways first class passenger Paul Trinder, who awoke "to find cabin crew had placed a corpse in his row without saying a word" (Schneider, 2014, p. 2). Apparently, it is common for crewmembers to place a deceased passenger in an open seat, including first/business class seats. While the flight attendants had the best intentions and in most cases, covered the corpse with a blanket, this is not the way to encourage repeat airline business. Mr. Trinder described the deceased passenger next to him, "she kept slipping under the seatbelt and moving about with the motion of the plane. When I asked what was going on, I was shocked to hear she was dead" (Schneider, 2014, p. 2). While a death in-flight is a rare occurrence, it is best to handle these infrequent emergencies with dignity for the deceased while minimizing the worry to passengers.

10-3-1-1. Airline In-Flight Death Policies

Off-duty EMS professionals shall check with crewmembers regarding the airline's policies in dealing with deceased passengers. Airline policies regarding in-flight deaths will vary, keep in mind that because deaths on-board aircraft are so rare, an on-board death may be the first death the crew has handled.

10-3-1-2. Storage of Body and "Corpse Cupboards"

When the death is unwitnessed and a body is discovered in its assigned seat, consult with the crewmembers on the procedure for storage of the body. The most logical location to store a deceased passenger is where it will be out of view from the other passengers, many times this will be in the aft (rear) galley. To prevent movement in-flight within the galley, a stored body shall be covered and wedged against a wall with blankets (Gabel et al., 2011). Other areas that may allow for the storage of a deceased passenger include 1) empty rows of seats away from passengers and 2) crew quarters on larger aircraft. There have been some reports that the deceased may be placed in an aircraft lavatory but current airline practices believe this is not ideal. Current airline training indicates:

> "You cannot put a dead passenger in the toilet. It's not respectful and [the corpse] is not strapped in for landing. If they slid off the toilet, they would end up on the floor. You would have to take the aircraft apart to get that person out. Imagine putting someone in the aircraft toilet" (Schneider, 2014, p. 2).

Larger wide-body aircraft may have designated storage areas suitable for corpses. Singapore Airlines carries body bags on certain aircraft and the airline's Airbus A340-500 planes were reported to be equipped with "corpse cupboards" for the storage of deceased passengers (Schneider, 2014, p. 2). After researching the "corpse cupboards" storage option, it has been determined that Singapore Airlines no longer utilizes this type of storage. In 2013, Singapore Airlines retired all Airbus A340-500's from their fleet and simultaneously retired the "corpse cupboards."

10-3-2. DIVERT WHEN POSSIBLE FOR DECEASED PASSENGER

Certain airlines choose to divert when possible in the event of a deceased passenger. Virgin Blue's procedure regarding in-flight deaths is to get on the ground as soon as possible to remove the corpse (Schneider, 2014). Lufthansa, on the other hand, believes that if a passenger is already dead, there is no medical urgency and a diversion is not recommended (Gabel et al., 2011). When unsure if a flight should be diverted for a deceased passenger, request consultation with a MedLink or ground-based physician for additional assistance. Additionally, if questioned by other passengers, it is best to be truthful when addressing the death of an on-board passenger.

10-3-3. RELIGIOUS CONSIDERATIONS OF THE DECEASED

When family and/or loved ones are traveling with the passenger who dies in-flight, notify them of the crewmember's intentions regarding the relocation of the deceased prior to moving the body. By notifying the family and loved ones, this may avoid any complications related to religious beliefs and customs. Make every attempt to work with the family of the deceased to resolve any unforeseen conflicts, if possible, when storing the deceased. Additionally, it may be determined that the continuation of the flight to its original destination (rather than diversion) is best for the family especially if religious beliefs require burial within 24 hours.

10-3-4. DO NOT STORE BODY NEXT TO UNAWARE PASSENGERS

If a decision has been made to place a deceased passenger in an empty seat or row, advise all the passengers within the immediate area and get acknowledgement from those passengers and when possible, allow those passengers to relocate to a different portion of the aircraft. If a passenger is deceased and already in a seat, it may be safer to leave the deceased passenger in their assigned seat. An aircraft that is being diverted to a closer airport for immediate removal of the deceased passenger should have their crew consider leaving the body as-is in their assigned seat for safety. Moving a body (when not necessary) throughout a cabin can cause back and other lifting injuries to the off-duty EMS professionals, passengers, and crewmembers.

10-4. AIRLINES ARE REQUIRED TO REPORT IN-FLIGHT DEATHS

Since deceased persons must be reported to local authorities so death certificates may be issued, airlines around the globe are required to report these incidents. According to local regulations and laws, airlines must advise relevant authorities such as police, airport EMS, and the local coroner when a death occurs in-flight. Airlines that have on-board fatalities related to in-flight accidents and/or turbulence, are also required to report these incidents to the National Transportation Safety Board (NTSB) or appropriate agency for investigation. In addition to the requirements above, FAA reporting regulations require that U.S. registered aircraft report the following information:

1) Number of persons who died in-flight or were declared dead upon landing
2) The age of the deceased
3) Cause of death if known
4) If the aircraft was diverted
5) Equipment used to help care for the person (House of Representatives, 1998)

Chapter Notes

Chapter Notes

INDEX

REFERENCES

Airbus. (2015). *A380 dimensions & key data*. Retrieved from Airbus.com: http://www.airbus.com/aircraftfamilies/passengeraircraft/a380family/specifications/

Alves, D. P. (2015, February 27). MedAire Global Medical Director, Aviation Health. (A. Chase, Interviewer)

ANA Group. (2016, May 26). *ANA to Introduce 'ANA Doctor On Board Service'*. Retrieved from ANA: http://www.ana.co.jp/group/en/pr/pdf/20160526.pdf

Banyan. (2017, March 14). *Aviation Medicine*. Retrieved from Banyan STAT KIT: https://www.statkit.com/Aviation

Bashir, T. (2014). Patients crash more than airlines: A medical emergency. *Journal of Community Hospital Internal Medicine Perspectives, 4*(3). doi:10.3402/jchimp.v4.24730

Blakema, T. C., Branson, R. D., Britton, T., Eggert, J., Ortiz, H., & Rodriquez, D. (2014). Managing endotracheal tube cuff pressure at altitude: A comparison of four methods. Journal of Trauma Acute Care Surgery, 77(3), S240-S244. doi:10.1097/TA.0000000000000339

Brennan, T. (2013). In-flight 911: Airlines rely on Arizona buisness for help. *Fox 10 Phoenix*. Retrieved from http://www.fox10phoenix.com/story/23975722/2013/11/14/med-air

Buchanan, I., Duong, D., Katzer, R. J., Memmer, A., & Weber, M. (2014). Management of in-flight medical emergencies: Are senior medical students prepared to respond to this community need? *Western Journal of Emergency Medicine, XV*(7), 925-929. doi:10.5811/westjem.2014.9.22569

Campbell, P. M. (2007). *Manual of in-flight medical care* (2nd ed.). Tempe: Kendall/Hunt Publishing Company.

Chandra, A., & Conry, S. (2013). In-flight medical emergencies. *Western Journal of Emergency Medicine, XIV*(5), 499-504. doi:10.5811/westjem.2013.4.16052

Cocks, R., & Liew, M. (2007). Commercial aviation in-flight emergencies and the physician. *Emergency Medicine Australasia, 19*, 1-8. doi:10.1111/j.1742-6723.2006.00928.x

Davis, R., & DeBarros, A. (2008). In the air, health emergencies rise quietly. *USA Today*. Retrieved from http://usatoday30.usatoday.com/news/health/2008-03-11-inflight-medical-emergencies_N.htm

European Aviation Safety Industry. (2015). *The Agency*. Retrieved from European Aviation Safety Agency: http://easa.europa.eu/the-agency

Federal Aviation Administration. (2006). *Advisory Circular No: 121-33B*. Retrieved from http://www.faa.gov/documentLibrary/media/Advisory_Circular/AC121-33B.pdf

Federal Aviation Administration. (2006). *Advisory circular No: 121-34B*. Retrieved from http://www.faa.gov/regulations_policies/advisory_circulars/index.cfm/go/document.information/documentID/22519

Gabel, A., Gebhard, J., Kaul, G., Muller-Rostin, W., Mulmann, M. V., & Stuben, U. (2011). *Handbook of aviation medicine and inflight medical emergencies.* Berlin: Medizinisch Wissenschaftliche Verlagsgesellschaft Berlin.

Glover, C. (2010). Medical emergency at 30,000 feet. *Nursing, 40*(9), 42-54. doi:10.1097/01.NURSE.0000387154.85491.2b

Graf, J., Stuben, U., & Pump, S. (2012, September 14). In-flight medical emergencies. *Deutsches Arzteblatt International, 109*(37), 591-602. doi:10.3238/arztebl.2012.0591

Harrison, K. J. (2006). MedAire expanding beyond medical expertise for travelers. *Aviation International News*. Retrieved from http://www.ainonline.com/aviation-news/aviation-international-news/2006-11-06/medaire-expanding-beyond-medical-expertise-travelers

Hordinsky, J., & George, M. (1991). *Utilization of emergency kits by air carriers.* Washington, D.C.: Office of Aviation Medicine; U.S. Department of Transportation; Federal Aviation Administration.

House of Representatives. (1998). *Aviation medical assistance act of 1998.* 105th Congress, 2d Session. Retrieved from http://www.gpo.gov/fdsys/pkg/CRPT-105hrpt456/pdf/CRPT-105hrpt456.pdf

ICAO. (2017, March 19). *Operation of Aircraft, Part 1, Chapter 6, Attachment B - Medical Supplies.* Retrieved from ICAO Health-Related Doccuments: http://www.icao.int/MID/Documents/2013/capsca-mid3/ICAOHealthRelatedSARPsandguidelines.pdf#search=Universal%20Precaution%20Kit

Joint Aviation Authorities. (2009). *Introduction to the JAA*. Retrieved from The European Joint Aviation Authorities: http://www.jaa.nl/introduction/introduction.html

Kovac, C. (1999). Airline passenger dies afterbeing sedated by doctor. *British Medical Journal, 18*, 12. doi:http://dx.doi.org.ezaccess.libraries.psu.edu/10.1136/bmj.318.7175.12b

Liao, M. (2010). Handiling in-flight medical emergencies. *Journal of Emergency Medical Services*. Retrieved from http://www.jems.com/articles/2010/06/handling-flight-medical-emerge.html

Lufthansa. (2015). *The 'Doctor on board' programme*. Retrieved from Lufthansa.com: http://www.lufthansa.com/us/en/Doctor-on-board

Lufthansa Group. (2015, 01 06). *A flying intensive care unit on all long-hual routes.* Retrieved from Lufthansa Media Relations: https://www.lufthansagroup.com/en/press/news-releases/singleview/archive/2015/june/01/article/3525.html

Lufthansa Medical Service, F. a. (2012, 09 14). *In-Flight Medical Emergencies Photo*. Retrieved 03 05, 2017, from Google: https://www.aerzteblatt.de/bilder/cache/00/00/05/27/img-52788-250-0.JPG

Lufthansa. (n.d.). *Patient Transport Compartment (PTC).* Retrieved from http://www.lufthansa.com/online/portal/lh/us/info_and_services/partner?nodeid=1653250719&l=en

MedAire. (2014). *Home*. Retrieved from MedAire an international SOS company: http://www.medaire.com/

MedAire. (2014). *Medical Advisory Services: MedLink*. Retrieved from MedAire.com: http://www.medaire.com/solutions/airlines/solutions/medical-advisory-services-medlink

MedAire Inc. (2017, March 17). Various MedAire Product Photographs . *Permission to Use Photographs by Director of Product Marketing, Mandy Eddington*. Phoenix, AZ, USA.

National Oceanic and Atmosphere Administration. (2015). *Air traffic with day/night terminator.* Retrieved from http://sos.noaa.gov/Datasets/dataset.php?id=44

O'Rourke, M. F., Donaldson, E., & Geddes, J. S. (1997). An airline cardiac arrest program. *The American Heart Association Journals*(96), 2849-2853. doi:10.1161/01.CIR.96.9.2849

Page, R. L., Joglar, J. A., Kowal, R. C., Kagrodzky, J., Nelson, L. L., ..., & McKenan, D. K. (2000). Use of automated external defibrillators by U.S. airline. *The New England Journal of Medicine*(343), 1210-1216. doi:10.1056/NEJM200010263431702

Peterson, D. C., Martin-Gill, C., Guyette, F. X., Tobias, A. Z., McCarthy, C. E., ..., & Yealy, D. M. (2013). Outcomes of medical emergencies on commercial airline flights. *The New England Journal of Medicine*(368), 2075-2083. doi:10.1056/NEJMoa1212052

Rahim Valani, M. C. (2010). Flight diversions due to onboard medical emergencies on an international commercial airline. *Aviation, Space, and Environmental Medicine*, 1037-1040.

Roach, B., Echols, K., & Burnett, a. A. (2014). *Excited Delirium and the Dual Response*. Retrieved from Federal Bureau of Investigation: http://leb.fbi.gov/2014/july/excited-delirium-and-the-dual-response-preventing-in-custody-deaths

Rushkin, K. J., Hernandez, K. A., & Barash, P. G. (2008). Management of in-flight medical emergencies. *Anesthesiology, 108*(4), 749-755.

Sand, M., Bechara, F.-G., Sand, D., & Mann, B. (2009). Surgical and medical emergencies on board European aircraft: a retrospective study of 10189 cases. *Critical Care, 13*(1), 1-6. doi:10.1186/cc7690

Sand, M., Morrosch, S., Sand, D., Altmeyer, P., & Bechara, F. G. (2012). Medical emergencies on board commercial airlines: is documentation as expected? *Critical Care*(16), 01-07. doi:10.1186/cc11238

Schneider, K. (2014). *What really happens when someone dies on a plane?* Retrieved from News.com.au: http://www.news.com.au/travel/travel-updates/what-really-happens-when-someone-dies-on-a-plane/story-fnizu68q-1226936994935

Silverman, D., & Gendreau, M. (2008). Medical issues associated with commercial flights. *The Lancet*(373), 2067-77. doi:10.1016/S0140-6736(09)60209-9

Sirven, J. I. (2006). *Is there a neurologist on this flight?* Retrieved from Universities Space Research Association: http://www.dsls.usra.edu/20060926.pdf

State EMS agency information. (2015). Retrieved from National registry of Emergency Medical Technitions: https://www.nremt.org/nremt/about/emt_cand_state_offices.asp

Stewart, P. H., Agin, W. S., & Douglas, S. (2013). What does the law say to good samaritans? A review of good samaritan statutes in 50 states and on US airlines. *Medical Ethics, 143*(6), 1774-1783.

Stocke, I. (2015, March 05). Commercial Airline Pilot, 1st Officer. (A. Chase, Interviewer)

Stone, M. D., Lubarsky, D. A., & Agarwal, G. G. (2014). Lessions learned during an in-flight medical emergency; Case report and discussion. *Journal of Travel Medicine*, 130-132. doi:10.1111/jtm.12087

The First Call. (2015). *Our services, Delivering in-flight medical advice globally* . Retrieved from The First Call; International Centre for International Medicine: http://www.thefirstcall.com/air/

Thompson, C. A. (2015). Know whats in airplane emergency medical kit, Two pharmacists say. *ASHP*. Retrieved from http://www.ashp.org/menu/News/PharmacyNews/NewsArticle.aspx?id=4158

Tobias, M. W. (2013). What happens if you become seriously ill during a flight. *Forbes*. Retrieved from http://www.forbes.com/sites/marcwebertobias/2013/01/22/what-happens-if-you-become-seriously-ill-during-a-flight/

Turkish Airlines. (2017, January). *Smiling Doctors*. Retrieved from Miles&Smiles: https://p.turkishairlines.com/en-us/miles-and-smiles/news/index.html

U. S. Government Publishing Office. (2015a). *CFR 121.333 Supplemental oxygen for emergency decent and for first aid.* Retrieved from Electronic Code of Federal Regulations: http://www.ecfr.gov/cgi-bin/text-idx?node=14:3.0.1.1.7.11.2.24&rgn=div8

U. S. Government Publishing Office. (2015b). *Part 121- operagting requirements: Domestic, flag, and supplemental operations.* Retrieved from http://www.ecfr.gov/cgi-bin/text-idx?c=ecfr&sid=3a80f64566bcc4375d9bd11aa85047be&rgn=div5&view=text&node=14:3.0.1.1.7&idno=14#se14.3.121_1333

U.S. Government Publishing Office. (2015c). *121.803 Emergency Medical Equipment.* Retrieved from Electronic code of federal regulations: http://www.ecfr.gov/cgi-bin/text-idx?SID=553d8fa2680ce1495de7fa4e5f69a10a&mc=true&node=se14.3.121_1803&rgn=div8

U.S. Government Publishing Office. (2015d). *Appendix to Part 121.* Retrieved from Electronic Code of Federal Regulations: http://www.ecfr.gov/cgi-bin/text-idx?SID=1357dcea68063daa2ea788abfa5d7ac4&mc=true&node=ap14.3.121_11500.a&rgn=div9

University of Pittsburgh. (2013). *'Is There a Doctor On Board?' Travelers Play Valuable Role Assisting Crew in Common Medical Emergencies on Flights.* Retrieved from UPMC: http://www.upmc.com/media/NewsReleases/2013/Pages/travelers-play-role-assisting-crew-in-medical-emergencies-on-flight.aspx

Zhang, B. (2016, 04 07). Crazy facts about planes that airline workers won't tell you. *Business Insider*, p. 7. Retrieved from http://www.businessinsider.com/airplane-curious-oxygen-rat-lavatory-2016-4